50 CARBS
2015 English Edition

by
José Quintana
with
Michael Calderwood

50 Carbs
Los Angeles, California

50 Carbs 2015 English Edition
Copyright © 2015
José Quintana and Michael Calderwood

All rights reserved. This book or any portion thereof may not be reproduced or used in any manner whatsoever without the express written permission of the publisher except for the use of brief quotations in a book review.
Printed in the United States of America
Updated April 2015
ISBN 978-0-9862720-3-5
50 Carbs Books
www.50Carbs.com

On the cover – a representation of one day's menu of meals and snacks that deliver delicious satisfaction – for 50 Carbs.

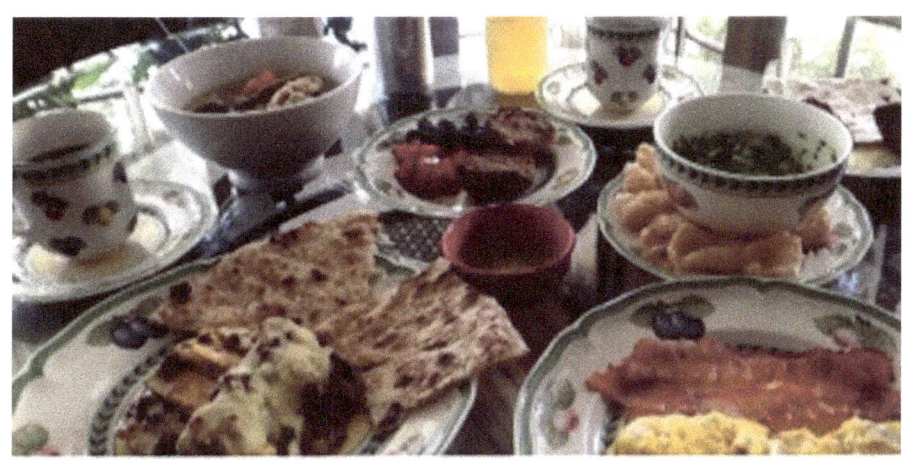

50 Carbs – it just makes sense!

Fher Olvera, *Philanthropist, Lead Singer for Maná*

"Seeing his transformation and hearing his story was inspiring, and showed me that there are ways to make positive changes in our life. I know so many people – friends, family and fans alike, who would find help, guidance and inspiration in Pepé's story. With obesity and diabetes high on the health concerns chart, the 50 Carbs plan that transformed my friend should find a place in every home, everywhere."

Dr. Michael Marsh, *Physician*

The "50 Carb" approach makes good sense, and goes after the key obstacles - hunger and boring meals – that cause many well-intentioned diet regimens to eventually fail. This sensible, managed approach to health and diet can be a great game plan for anyone who has been struggling to take charge of their own health. I am so pleased to see the change in José, and would be equally pleased to see these changes in everyone who suffers the sad effects of poor diet."

Michael Calderwood, *co-author 50 Carbs*

I first met José at a very happy time for both of us - our kids were getting married! We quickly became friends and family. We both love music and bad jokes - you might say we are experts at one or the other!

As José started his journey to what has become 50 Carbs, I saw a real strength and determination that was both impressive and inspiring. When he suggested sharing his story I knew I wanted to be part of it. It became our goal to tell this story in a way that would give help and inspiration to others who struggle with the problems that come with poor diet. In the end, 50 Carbs is the story of José's search and ultimate success in finding a low-stress, healthy and practical plan to manage his weight.

50 CARBS	1
ME	3
THE WAKEUP	16
MY BODY	18
STARTING THE JOURNEY	21
GETTING ORGANIZED	23
STRATEGY	25
CARBS…	27
TOOLS	29
THE FIRST WEEKS	34
BREAKFAST	37
SNACKS	42
LUNCH AND DINNER	51
COOKWARE	58
OUT AND ABOUT	64
QUICK NOTES…	68
PREPARE FOR TAKEOFF	71
SHORT CUTS	76
GO GET IT!	81
ONE YEAR LATER	85
NO APP?	90
MAINTENANCE MODE	96
FROM A FRIEND	101
FROM MY DOCTOR	103
JOSÉ	105

50 Carbs

Diabetes. High blood pressure. High cholesterol. Low energy. Too much weight. Bigger clothes. Poor sleep. Not the happiest of words to see and hear when you're thinking of your health. And especially when a lot of them are coming from your doctor.

These were the words that described what I had let myself become. Years of bad habits, bad information, and bad food choices got me into bad shape. I only had to open my medicine cabinet to see the results of all that bad. A lineup of medications designed to slow down the march towards disaster. They helped but still…

I got tired of being tired. I got really tired of hearing those words. I got really *really* tired of looking in my medicine cabinet. Now, I could get a new medicine cabinet, or I could clean out the old one. See – I started making good choices!

Enter 50 Carbs. (Drumroll please!)

As you'll read in this book, I made a choice – get my health under control and change the things that were breaking me down. I spent a lot of time and energy researching, experimenting and ultimately designing a program that would be my guide – my personal health GPS. I knew what had caused me to get lost in previous trips through diet country, and I made sensible course corrections that got me to where I am today.

Now the words I hear from my doctor? Well, here's what he said after my last checkup.

"Jose, I hope you're sitting down… I want to read your book!... These numbers are FANTASTIC! … Blood sugar, cholesterol, blood pressure – down… I want you to come back in so we can start taking down your medicines. I don't think you need them anymore".

So, no more medicines. I am so skinny I have to stand in the same spot twice to make a shadow! Seriously, I am healthy, happy and ready for the next act in my great life story. I truly believe that anyone looking to break away from all the "bad" words will find help and success with the 50 Carbs plan. Please take it and make it your own. Let's get going!

Chapter 1
ME

In my soul, I am a musician.

My Early Days

Most of my childhood memories have been erased from my mind. I was the youngest of 9 brothers and sisters. I don't remember having the perception of us being a very united family. Pretty much everybody left home early to make their own lives. We kept little contact with each other.

From the very little that I know, my mother had my first brother at the age of 13. She was 40 when I was born.

My mother developed some kind of health condition. Her doctor advised her to live at sea level. This kept her away from me and unfortunately I didn't have the chance to see her much. The time when she decided to come and stay with us she suffered an aneurism and passed away.

My father worked for the Mexican railroad system as a Station Manager. We would spend a couple of years in a town somewhere in the country before we would have to move to another town, in another state. All of my brothers and sisters were born in different towns in Mexico.

One of my sisters helped to raise me. She did what she could but she had her own dreams to pursue. She was an accomplished classical pianist. I remember her practicing scales or classical pieces for 10 hours a day. All day long the sound of music filled our house.

One day her teacher asked me if I would like to learn to play the piano. I said yes! It was then, at the age of five when I discovered my passion for music. Since then it has been my life.

My earliest memory of performing was at the age of 6. I played a recital of classical music (appropriate for my age) at the "Sala Chopin," a very prestigious music hall in Mexico City.

A few years later my beloved father succumbed to diabetes. This disease would follow me throughout my life.

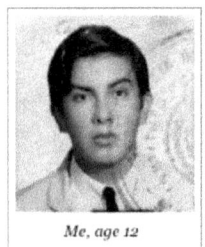
Me, age 12

So, by the time I became a teenager I had lost both my parents. I had to find a way to make a living, and a way to make my dreams come true.

Music was that dream, so music was the path I followed.

I chose the bass guitar as my instrument. After a very rough beginning I progressed, little by little, to playing with Orquestas, Rock Bands, and Top 40 bands. I was able to find gigs as a recording session player, play in a TV house band, play on tours - anything that had to do with live music. I was making my living as a musician.

The 1960's

I had a great time.

One of my best memories is from the early 60's. I was around 14 years old, and a "groupie" of a popular rock band in Mexico called "Los Rebeldes del Rock." They got booked to play an important wedding in Mexicali (a three day trip by bus from Mexico City). Me and a bunch of guys went to the bus station to wish them a good trip.

The bus was ready to depart but the band's bass player was missing. The bandleader knew that I played bass and asked me to jump on the bus and be the bass player for that particular event!

50 Carbs

Well, I had nobody at home I had to report to, so I jumped on that bus with only the clothes I had on. Before I could reach my seat the bus took off. I was on my way to Mexicali!

We arrived in Mexicali a few days early so we decided to go to Tijuana, which was considered the mecca for Mexican Rock bands. There were a few clubs that featured really great live music.

"Mikes" was one of the most popular clubs. When we went in the house bandleader recognized our band and asked us to play a set (a palomazo). We played, and the reaction was so fantastic that the owner hired us for 3 months.

Mexico City

We came back to Mexico City 4 months later. Shortly after my return I joined the house band of a "vaudeville" type of nightclub called Terraza Casino. Our job was to back up all the artists that were part of the show. The job was a little strong for a 15 year-old boy, but being surrounded all night by lots of girls in small bikinis made the job not too painful. I suffered this job for over a year!

From there I joined a band called "The Loud Jets" and for 8 years we found good gigs. Instead of being a pure rock band we were playing International Music.

Did I mention I had a great time? Perhaps not much money was available but the job had great perks. We loved those "3 month gigs" at a luxury resort somewhere in the world. We were always allowed to get good accommodations, and fabulous food was plentiful and free of charge for the band.

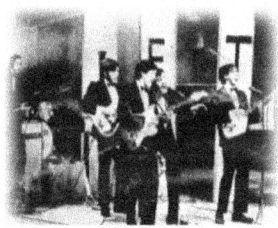
The Loud Jets. José Quintana on bass, second from left.

During the last 4 years of my life in Mexico we landed a steady job at "Restaurant Del Lago," one of the best restaurants in Mexico City. I became very friendly with the chef, and every night I had (under the table) the most incredible gourmet dinners.

5

As you can tell I became very spoiled, especially regarding food! Little by little my stomach started to grow, but it was impossible for me to say no these daily feasts.

If I had to decide between my waistline or magnificent food, I always went for the food.

Los Angeles bound

1970's - 1980's

I moved to the USA in the late 70's. After a very rough beginning that lasted a bit over a year, things turned around and my career quickly took off. Before I knew it I was managing and producing or co-producing the recordings of the main superstars of Latin America.

Besides the creative stuff, my work description involved hosting the artists while they were in Los Angeles recording. All these Superstars from Mexico, Spain, Argentina, Miami and other places came to record with me for 1 to 4 months.

Some of them had never been to L.A. before so I would meet them at the airport and take them to one of the 5 - star hotels. I had to take them out to eat their 3 daily meals in first class restaurants (a good bonding moment for me with them). And I always had to take them to Disneyland - over 20 times in 18 months!

Due to the stature of the artist we always worked in top of the line recording studios. These great facilities always try to make your life as pleasant as possible, and food was one of the items that was always present.

We'd arrive at 10 in the morning and there was a big basket filled with pastries, donuts, fruit, cheese, bagels, coffees and juices waiting for us.

By eleven we'd order a coffee run - vanilla latte, cappuccinos, espressos…

Around noon the client services people would ask what we were going to eat for lunch. After looking in a book with menus from hundred of places, we'd choose what we wanted and send one of the runners to get it. The order could be anything from a simple sandwich to a really elaborate dish (Chinese, Mexican, Italian, steaks, ribs, fries, potato salad, coleslaw, milk shakes, cake).

By 6 PM the studio people had baked chocolate chip cookies for us and sent the runner on another coffee run.

By ten PM we'd finish our session for the day, and it was time for dinner at one of LA's happening clubs or restaurants.

My clients always wanted to go to the most exciting places, and they usually ordered big. After all, it was "free." The record companies would cover their expenses for food, lodging and entertainment while they were in town recording (ah, the good old days!). The biggest of these superstars had unlimited budgets, so why not take advantage of it? I never had trouble getting reimbursed by the record companies for food and entertainment.

That was my daily routine for two years. Now picture me when I had 2 or 3 projects overlapping and I had to eat double! All that great (but oh so rich) food I was consuming was starting to create the layer of dense fat that I carried for the next 30 years.

It was also nesting my diabetes.

A&M Records

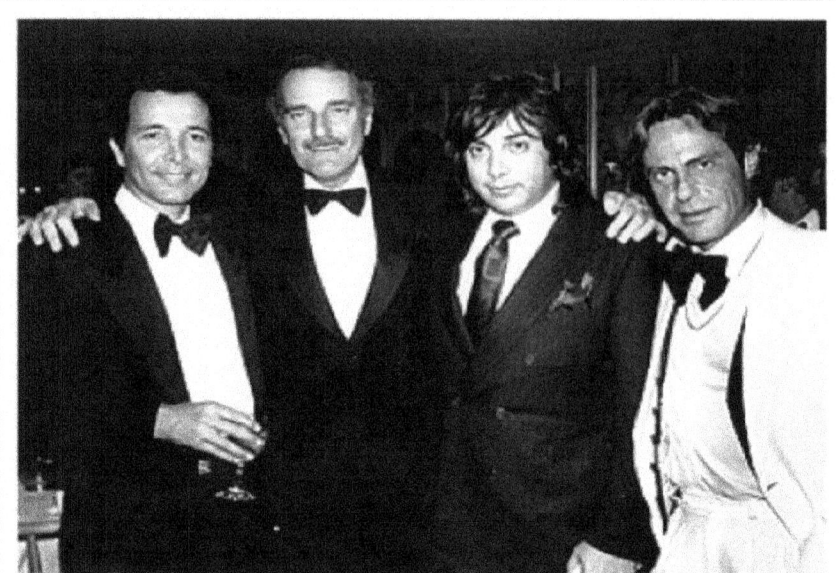

Legendary founders of A&M Records Herb Alpert and Jerry Moss with Jose Quintana and composer/musician Juan Carlos Calderon at the 1982 A&M Grammy party.
  Photo courtesy of Sam Emerson

For the next 8 years I worked for one of the biggest and most successful global record companies of the 1980's – A&M Records – running their Latin Division. What a great time I had there! The Christmas parties were legendary, with over 200 employees filling their Los Angeles headquarters. With a cost of well over six figures, you can be sure the food was exceptionally good.

In addition to looking after the business side of the Latin division, I was responsible for finding artists for the roster. I had a busy schedule filled with breakfasts, lunches and dinners with artists, managers, writers, publishers, music attorneys, producers, arrangers and international affiliates. I also had to make frequent trips to the East Coast, Mexico, South America, Spain and Italy. I had a company credit card for my expenses. I took limos, traveled First Class, and stayed in the best hotels.

It's interesting to see how much of my business was conducted over a meal. I think I sponsored over 300 Los Angeles restaurants in the big 80's. You would find me doing my thing at places like Ma Maison, The Palm, Citrus, Mr. Chow, LeDome, Lawry's, Gardel's, The Ivy, La loggia, Muse, Au Petite, La Boheme, Chasen's and Benihana.

When visiting our overseas affiliates I was treated like royalty, eating in the best restaurants of Madrid, Barcelona, Buenos Aires, Rio, Mexico City, and Guadalajara.

I wouldn't know how to begin describing all the great food I consumed during this period. I can say for sure that I experienced hundreds of meals that reached "food ecstasy" status.

I dieted many times in the 80's. I had periods where I let myself go, and I ballooned to over 200 pounds. There were times I would lower my weight to 180 pounds. It was a constant battle.

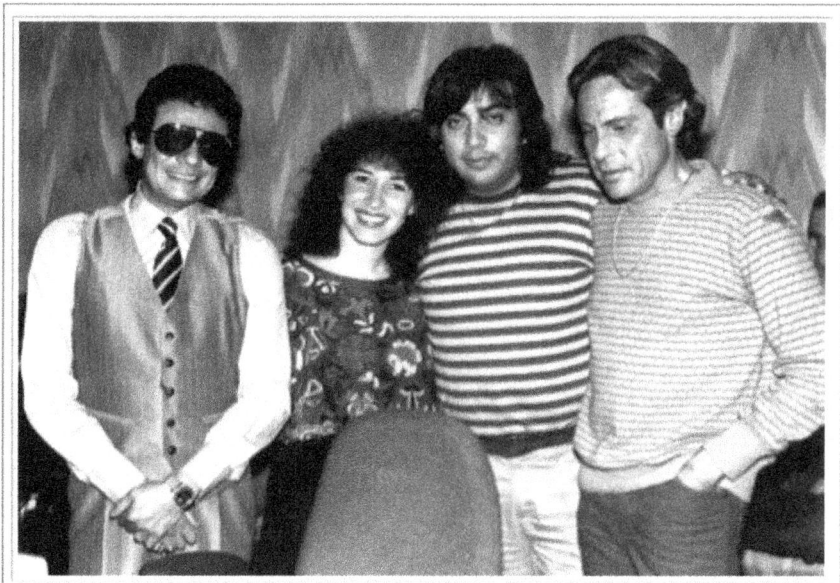

Recording session for Lani Hall's Grammy-winning Best Latin Album. With Jose Jose, Lani Hall, Jose Quintana and Juan Carlos Calderon. Jose Jose was considered the "Frank Sinatra of Latin America."
Photo courtesy of Patty McKenna

The 1990'S

The 90's. A new decade, and a new job. I moved to Warner Brothers Mexico, taking on similar duties with that label. The perks were pretty much the same, too. The job did require one major change, though. I needed to spend 5 days a week in Mexico City, with weekends back home in Los Angeles.

So here I am in Mexico City, my "food paradise". This world-famous food is so good, and if you know where to go it is really hard to resist. Besides the thousands of gourmet restaurants in the city, the street food cannot be surpassed by any other, anywhere. The canasta sweaty tacos, the taco stands, the "fondas" – little restaurants in the food markets – everything made with fresh raw ingredients and open for business 24/7. So I ate.

More Changes

Traveling to Mexico every week for 2 years was getting too crazy for me, so I decided to quit and try the independent life as a producer or production manager.

I got involved right away in a few important recordings where budgets were pretty much unlimited.

The recording of an album took an average of 3 months. I remember approving around $8000 in charges just in coffee runs. The food charges were way more. Our staff of up to 8 people ate very well, enjoying meals delivered from the best restaurants in the Hollywood area.

Coast to Coast

A couple of years later I got hired by Sony Latin, based in Miami. Although my responsibilities required me to find talent on the west coast of the USA I also had to travel to Miami a few times a month.

Authentic Mexican food was mainly targeted for the millions of

50 Carbs

Mexican consumers that live in what's known as "Mex-America," a loose belt running from California to Texas to Mexico, with food and product stands on every other corner of the main cities.

In Florida a similar cultural flavor rules, only with Cuban food. It seems that they love bread as much as I do! There is a popular sandwich called "torta cubana" made with a toasted and buttered Cuban bread (large baguette) stuffed with ham, Swiss cheese, roast pork and mustard. They also make all kinds of great pork and steak sandwich variations with this type of bread.

This easy-to-find Cuban bread is also very popular for breakfast. It's heavily buttered and toasted in a panini machine, and enjoyed with a cup of one of the many strong Cuban coffees. That's a tasty treat and most of the time it's enough to give you the jolt you need to get you going in the morning.

There is an old Cuban restaurant in Miami called "Versailles" that has a special place in my heart for the memorable meals I had there. Dishes like Paella, Ropa Vieja, Zarsuela de mariscos, Roast Pork Cuban Style, Milanesa, Moros rice (rice and beans) and dozens of more tasty dishes on the menu. Just thinking about it makes my mouth watery.

Miami is the closest place in United States to connect to every country in North, Central and South America. There are hundreds of fantastic restaurants featuring the full range of Latin cuisine - dishes from Argentina, Peru, Chile, Colombia and Central America. So many of these dishes are just spectacular.

The Century Turns

The turn of the century brought some drastic changes to my life. New technologies brought major changes to the recording industry, and affected the fields I depended on. The growth in music piracy contributed to the decline of the music business that I knew and was a part of all my life.

All those big-budget recording sessions ended. No more company credit cards to wave at those expensive meals. A few cycles of unemployment pushed me to make a few changes; if I wanted to continue to please my spoiled palate I had to learn how the food I loved was prepared. I began to ask and learn from people who knew and understood how to cook well.

During this time of transition I was very blessed to work with Maná, one of the most popular bands in Latino America. A few of the recordings I was involved with took me away from home for a few months. Every time they recorded an album, we'd set up a studio to record the lead vocals in a very inspiring location in Puerto Vallarta.

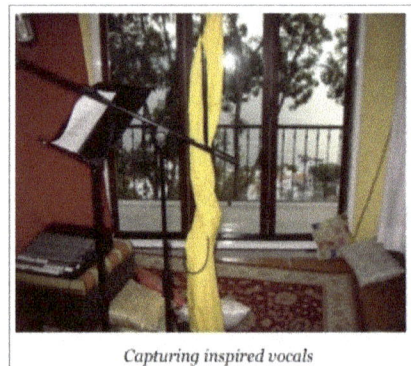

Capturing inspired vocals

They would rent a villa up in the hills, with a dramatic view of the coastline - a must for singing inspiration. The house was professionally staffed with a very efficient team that included chefs that prepared breakfast, lunch, dinner and snacks all day for 4 people.

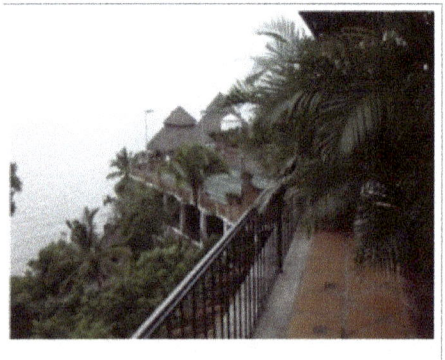

The view from the balcony

Lessons Learned

I remember one of these recording sessions we did in 2010. We had a chef named Julio, who was amazingly talented. He would surprise us every day with the most incredible meals, which included a picture-taking presentation. I enjoyed every meal he prepared.

Julio and I became good friends. He knew I was curious about cooking, and that I wanted to learn how to prepare a decent meal for myself at home. He shared some of his cooking knowledge with me.

Julio gave me some great advice and taught me a lot of the cooking basics. I went to the market with him a few times to get the ingredients for the day's dishes. Watching him go through the piles of fruits and vegetables taught me not to be fooled by the biggest piece on the pile, but rather pick normal-sized items. He told me that the larger items might look good, but the flavor often gets diluted.

He believed that one of the main factors in making a dish taste good is learning how much stronger the flavors are rendered by the order you throw them into the pan. For instance if you are going to start your dish by frying onions and garlic, heat some oil in your pan. Once the pan is hot, throw the onions in first and fry them for a couple of minutes. Then add the garlic and cook together. Add salt and pepper, and it's ready before the garlic gets brown. If you want to add more ingredients like carrots, tomatoes, celery or peppers this is the moment to do it. Add them to your onion and garlic mixture, fry them until it looks cooked - you can tell when this mixture is done and is ready to enhance a lot of sauces, meats, soups and vegetables.

The next piece of advice he gave me was pretty simple, but absolutely critical. Allow enough time to cook your dishes. Don't rush or undercook them. When cooking meat do not flip it over and over; flip it only one time to cook the other side. Before serving let the meat rest for a few minutes. Do the same for casseroles or desserts. Not the flipping – the resting!

Another important lesson was learning to use the right cookware for my dishes, and how to use different cooking mediums to achieve the flavor, look, texture and taste I was looking for.

After this "cooking boot camp" I came home ready to start creating my own delicious meals with much better knowledge about how to do it right. From that point until now I have improved big time the flavor of my meals.

Julio's Tips

- *Take care to pick the best, not the biggest fruits and veggies*
- *Release the flavors at the right time, in the right order*
- *Don't flip out! One and done!*
- *Let the meat rest (but not loaf!)*
- *Cooking vessels - use the right tools for the job*
- *Use different methods for different meals.*
- *Be not afraid – of new flavors.*

Julio's Amazing Feasts

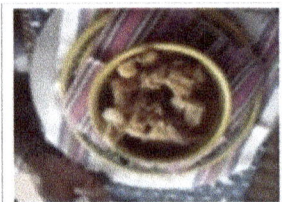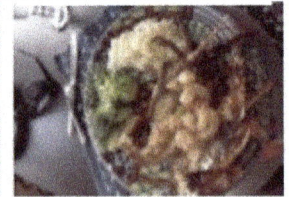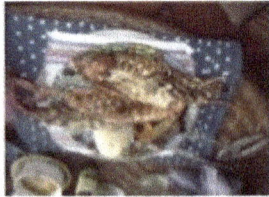

Seafood heaven with shrimp, lobster and magic!

Still Learning

I don't claim to be a chef (or even resemble one). I just learned the way to "correctly" prepare a few meals that worked for me and really pleased my palate. They were delicious, easy, fast and economical to make, using products that were in my pantry and easy to find in any market.

As you can guess, many of these meals were not carb conscious; there was plenty of stuff like pastas, rice, pastries and desserts in my repertoire.

As my professional music career was dimming I used lots of the free time I had on my hands to focus on the food topic. I cooked all kind of dishes and had to eat them all. No wonder I ballooned to 210 pounds!

When I look at pictures of me from the 6 years before writing this

50 Carbs

book I can see my progressive gain in size. Six months ago when I hit the 210-pound mark, my inner boy said "that's enough."

And so it went, until we arrive at the here and now.

Chapter 2

The Wakeup

Twelve years ago I was diagnosed with diabetes. Since then, I have been taking four different medications – twice a day – to control the disease. Twelve years, four medications, twice a day. (That is a lot of pills!)

My prescriptions would be automatically refilled every three months. A month before I started my diet, my pills were denied. The number of refills had been reached, and my doctor wanted to see me before he would renew them. It had been over a year since my last visit, and I needed to make the appointment soon.

This event triggered some kind of fear in me. I knew immediately that the first thing the doctor would order was a complete physical that included the A1C blood test. This test would paint a picture of my food intake behavior for the last 3 months. Heart function, cholesterol levels and blood pressure numbers would tell the story.

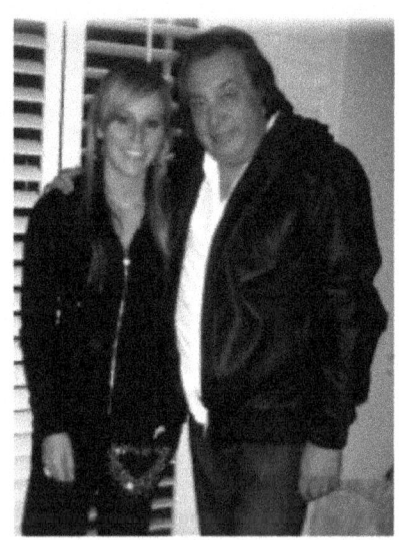
Jose and his daughter Heather, 2009

My lifestyle over the last couple of years before the doctor's visit made me feel that I was in trouble for sure. I was not very responsible about taking care of my body, and I was about to face the truth that I'd been evading for many years.

By then I was heavier than ever. I had plumped up to 210 lbs. I had not walked for years. My blood pressure and glucose readings were high, so naturally I anticipated very negative results.

A week later the results came back. I had no doubt that I was going to hear bad news, and I was very afraid to hear it. After waiting for a while I finally found some courage and I called my doctor to find out the results. It was a nerve- wracking moment.

I was overjoyed to hear that the results were not as bad as I anticipated. They were not good either, but from my perspective I strongly felt that I was at an important place.

If I was going to get serious about taking care of my abandoned body, I would have to re-route my life to a more positive, healthier lifestyle, and live my life from now until the end without carrying the many terrible medical problems that develop with diabetes. Perhaps this action could extend my life for a few more years.

It's a fact- the only way for anybody to lose weight is by starving your body. You have to drastically reduce your food intake to levels that the body needs to use your own fat to function. The same principle applies to all the diets.

What makes all diets eventually crash? Hunger - the sensation of food depravation - is perhaps the biggest enemy, followed by small portions of funny-tasting, unattractive food that we have to consume to lose the weight. Then comes the torture of keeping the weight off under this unpleasant life style. Not an easy task. Kind of a depressing way to live but this is the kind of sacrifice you need to make in order to enjoy a better life.

It doesn't have to be this way. I developed this plan with an eye on making it successful on all fronts. And again, I have to say how smooth and stress-free this ride has been for me. I truly believe it can be just as beautiful for you.

Chapter 3
My Body

MY BODY

This machine, created by the celestial powers, is my most important piece of equipment. I cannot exist without it.

This precious machine requires permanent maintenance to run properly. Keeping my body trim helps it to work with less stress and to last longer. The feeling of your body working well -what better gift can you give to yourself?

Think about a car. If I keep a close eye on the maintenance, service it and refresh the fluids every time it's due, it is going to run great and will likely last for a long time.

Monitoring all the critical levels - gas, oil, coolants, brake fluids, tire pressure – lets me and my technician know if something needs attention before it becomes a problem.

The body needs the same level of attention.

In my case I spent too many years totally ignoring the signals my body was sending me. I carried a chronic pear shape- a big stomach, a double chin. The excessive weight caused me to snore very loudly, which contributed to poor sleep for me (and anyone nearby!). These signals were indications that my body needed help. Instead of listening to these signals, I let things go, and allowed some vital parts to break down. Being diagnosed with Diabetes ten years ago underlined this reality. The potential consequences of this disease could not be ignored.

I tried many times to get rid of some of my excessive weight, but it became an impossible task.

50 Carbs

And then, one day (not too long ago) I confronted myself. There I was, moving through my sixties, worrying about my health and how my remaining years would be impacted by the terrible consequences of my diabetes. I had to do something to change the story. I had to own my health.

And so I did.

The first thing I needed to do to manage my diabetes was to lose weight. Thinking back on what worked, and what didn't work with previous diet attempts, I knew I needed a detailed food plan and a reliable method to track and manage it. I spent days carefully experimenting with different foods until I created a plan that would be up to the task.

Destiny- meet determination and strategy.

Going into my plan I knew – or thought I knew - that losing 40 pounds was absolutely impossible for me. I was going to be happy if I could drop around 20 pounds in six months.

This time all the stars aligned for me as I implemented my plan. Everything came together rather quickly and worked so well that I lost over 50 pounds in four months! A remarkable achievement for someone in my age group by anybody's standard.

By following my plan, it seemed like I suddenly found the key to the gate - the gate that was holding my extra weight. I was able to unlock that gate and bring my weight down.

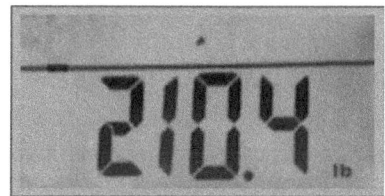 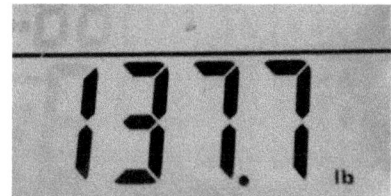

I went from 210.4 pounds down to 137.7 pounds – over 70 pounds. Over a quarter of my size in about 120 days.

The real blessing - one that I was not really expecting - was how comfortable the ride has been. Rather than "flying coach," I felt like I was flying First Class. The trip was the same – same time, same distance, same plane; the journey, however was smooth and practically stress free. A much better way to get me where I wanted – needed – to be.

The physical change that I made in such a short amount of time was so radical that many of my friends don't recognize me. Now, when they realize it's me, the flattering comments about my new look are non-stop. Everybody has the same comment : "It's inspiring!" And everybody wants to know how I did it.

I remember the comments of one of my best friends, who I had not seen in over 4 months. He said "Looking at you now, I see answers to important questions I had about how to help some of my overweight loved ones, friends and relatives. I believed they were doomed, and now I know there is hope because "if Pepe (me) did it at his age and life style, anybody can do it."

I can't help but smile when I see my new self in the mirror. It's so great for my psyche not to see the unflattering layers of fat that covered my body for most of my adult life. I am thrilled to have finally discovered the body that God meant for me. What a sublime experience.

Today a feeling of joy has invaded my life. I had never before experienced my body feeling this good. My whole system works without stress. It feels like my body is in "party" mode. I am happy, I am grateful, and I am celebrating this incredible feeling of success. It's the special kind of feeling you can only get from your own efforts. It is simply the best -- better than a Rolex, a car or a trip to Europe. It's hard to describe this sensation in words, but it is very profound.

I am still stunned over how easy my short journey was and the overwhelming results I got.

Chapter 4
Starting the Journey

THE NEW ROAD

My next step was to find a diet that would help me confront my number one enemy – HUNGER! I knew it would show up for the ride, trying to make my journey miserable. If I committed to improving my numbers, I would have to meet it face to face, and beat it every time.

From my past experience with weight loss I was familiar with how the most popular diets work, and what they offer. In my mind I classified them in two categories – Low Calorie Diets, and Low Carb Diets. Both regimens had worked fine for me; I think they work for anybody when the rules are strictly followed.

I usually started losing weight slowly. But for someone like me who loves food with a passion, the existence would soon become miserable. I would slip away, and then stop dieting all together. Hello again, weight gain!

I had to ask myself some tough questions. Which diet? Which one would be the least severe? Which one could I endure?

I found the low-calorie diet to be somewhat healthier than the low carb diet, but it was harder for me to stay with for longer than a couple of weeks. The food intake was very restricted, and all the ingredients that provide the delicious taste of fat to food disappears. Hello raw vegetables, goodbye yummy food!

The low carb diet can be pretty hard-core. After a few weeks of eating lots of meat, I started feeling both nauseous and clogged. Using meat as the largest component of my meals filled my plate, but also added some bad stuff to my system that could have been damaging if consumed in excess.

After researching and weighing the pros and cons of both approaches, I decided to go with the low carb diet. Even though it was over ten years ago, my experience with the Atkins Diet™, was still fresh in my mind. I knew what to expect. I remember I stayed on it for a while, and I slimmed down to around 180 pounds. I felt I conquered a big goal in my life. Then, little by little, I started leaving the diet. Before I knew it I was back where I started. And then some...

I gave up dieting, convincing myself that this was my destiny. I accepted that I would remain overweight forever. I believed there was nothing I could do about it. People in my age group couldn't take on this challenge. So I did nothing, not even the basic physical activity you need to keep moving. I just indulged myself, eating all kinds of foods without any restrictions. I loved food too much and my will power was very weak.

I did contemplate the possibility of removing the extra weight with surgeries such as tummy tuck, lap band or liposuction. They were not only very expensive and painful but didn't really address my main concern – managing the diabetes. I dropped this idea and decided to go the old fashioned way. After researching and weighing the pros and cons of both approaches, I decided to go with the low carb diet.

But...

I changed my mindset from weight loss to managing my diabetes. That became the priority. I figured if I lowered my glucose perhaps I'd drop a few pounds. That would be "the cherry on top." This simple but game-changing decision was <u>everything</u>. Relieving myself of the stress of trying to hit a weight-loss number and instead focusing of getting healthier changed my psychological outlook from fear to optimism. I would still need to meet and beat "hunger" and change my food-consuming ways. I felt that I was ready to face the music.

Chapter 5
Getting Organized

GETTING ORGANIZED

I realized that if I wanted to make this effort a success I would need to be well organized and disciplined. I needed to keep close track of my glucose numbers. During my Atkins days I would try to keep records, writing the numbers down on pieces of paper (when I remembered). After a while the information was scattered all over the place – different pieces of paper with bits of information, undated, unorganized and unusable. This time, I would keep a detailed, accurate daily record of my glucose numbers. I needed a tool that would help me do this.

I went on an internet search for an application that would give me what I needed. It had to be powerful enough to turn the data I entered into useful and easy to understand information. It needed to be self-contained and portable. I didn't want a repeat of my previous efforts. I wanted the app at my fingertips – to be where I was when I was eating. Since my smartphone is always close by, it made good sense to find an app that would run on a mobile platform.

I found there were many available that would allow me to enter my daily food intake and the associated carb values. These tools would keep me informed about my carb and calorie consumption at every meal. They also allowed me to enter the daily "out of bed" test results for the glucose levels that I that wanted to bring down from 150 mg to under 100 mg.

I spent a couple of days getting familiar with the app that I chose. The application was very intuitive – I learned how to enter and how to interpret the data in a few hours. The application was packed with information – there were over 200,000 food items in the databank so it got a little tricky to accurately enter the food items and portions that I was consuming at every meal. It is the most important thing to get right – accurate input will give accurate results. The app also had additional features that would let me track other important health components at the same time. I'll talk about them a bit later in the book.

I was ready to begin. I had a clear goal. I had an organized game plan. I had a tool that would let me accurately track my glucose numbers. I had a good diet strategy. I was ready to win.

Chapter 6
Strategy

THE PLAN

Once I understood how to negotiate my daily carb allowance, I began to focus on maximizing the appeal of each ingredient that went into each meal. My goal was to combat hunger by constantly supplying my body with "smart" food that can be easily found in any market.

I was able to prepare recipes using food that I loved, measuring the exact quantities so they did not exceed the carb budget. I used my special "Mexican Home Cooking" techniques, and most of my meals were quite enjoyable.

There are many low-carb products available in the market. If you can think of it, you can probably find just about anything. Some are really good, but boy can they get expensive. I didn't want to have a bigger grocery bill every week, and I wanted to include more fresh, natural foods in my plan. There were a few items I did use, but I really focused on creative exchanges.

I had to replace a couple of items from my old list of favorites like bread, tortillas, and sweets, and a few others. Thankfully there are good, easy to find substitute products that I could use to put back the rich flavors in my meals while still drastically reducing my carb intake!

Here's an example:

A typical Mexican carne asada taco using 2 corn tortillas has 55 grams of carbs (2 corn tortillas = 50 carbs, the rest of the ingredients combined are 5 grams)

I substituted low-carb tortillas, which have a carb value of 3 grams.

Strategy

This simple substitution saved me an amazing 47 grams of carbs! If I used one spoon of salsa instead of two, I saved an additional 1 gram. So one of my favorite meals went from 55 grams to 8 grams!

Now, the final results did not taste exactly the same as the original, but for me it was more than close enough to enjoy and keep me on plan.

There are many more examples like this. At first I thought that since I was in "diet mode" some of my meals would be less flavorful. By being creative in using herbs and spices, I was able to turn the flavor back on.

I had to be careful picking my food choices for the day. I had to give up or use only very small portions of some of my favorite side dishes like beans and rice. A couple of tablespoons of each cost me 8 grams of carbs or more; imagine the cost of a bowl!

This strategy was my main weapon in my fight against creeping hunger and deserves a lot of credit for the success of my weight loss journey. Unlike past diet attempts, this time my body never experienced the hunger pangs that used to make me crazy. Instead, my stomach felt satisfied most of the time.

The occasional waves of hunger I would feel during the program were what I would call the "tolerable kind." I never reached the point of "extreme hunger," and when I wanted to relieve these symptoms I would grab one of the many kinds of snacks I had prepared (and kept handy) to help ease the hunger and keep me on target. It is amazing how many healthy, delicious snack choices there are – literally hundreds.

I brought my passion for "Mexican Home Cooking" to my dishes. I had to make some changes to some ingredients to keep to my carb budget, but I was able to prepare delicious and satisfying food that helped me feel like I wasn't on a diet, but rather a tasty and satisfying journey to a slimmer, healthier me.

Chapter 7

Carbs...

What is a carbohydrate? Carbohydrates (carbs) are one of the three components in food that our body converts into energy and uses it to run.

The other two components are fats and amino acids. Carbohydrates turn to sugar, fat and amino acids that help in the creation of new cells.

Carbs According to Me!

• If you want to maintain your present weight, you have to limit your daily carbs consumption to 80 grams.

• If you want to start losing weight at a moderate pace, you have to limit your daily carb consumption to 50 grams; fewer if you want to lose weight quicker.

• If you want to lose weight very fast you have to go to 30 grams a day.

After experimenting with different targets I found 50 grams of carbs a day to be perfect for me.

I was happy to find so many good foods that I could cook myself. I could always have a decent meal, and I could keep track of the results with the help of my Smartphone and my Diabetes App.

I felt for the first time I had some control. There was no more guessing. I had solid, real information that told me where I stood at any time during the day. I knew this was powerful stuff that would take the fight out of my enemy - hunger!

The few times I did not follow the rules, the app on my phone would let me know. If I exceeded my carb budget, I was able to take steps to get back on plan. The corrections were easy, and over the course of a day or so I was back on target. No drama!

Calories

What is a calorie? A calorie is a measurement used for the amount of energy you consume through food.

The way I understand it is as if every day I'd inflate a tire and calories are like the gauge on the hose that tells me the amount of air I'm putting in that tire.

Remember, for my plan I focused on managing my carb intake. Of course, calories play a big role in weight management, and ignoring them is not a great idea. I factor the calories in to my overall approach to eating well, and I try to keep my daily caloric intake under 1500 per day. 1000 calories would be ideal.

I find the perfect balance of carbs and calories is like opening both faucets at the same time - getting benefits from both. I find that it is a bit easier to manage my weight more closely.

But again, my main focus, and the focus of this plan, is on carbs.

Chapter 8
Tools

TOOLS COUNT!

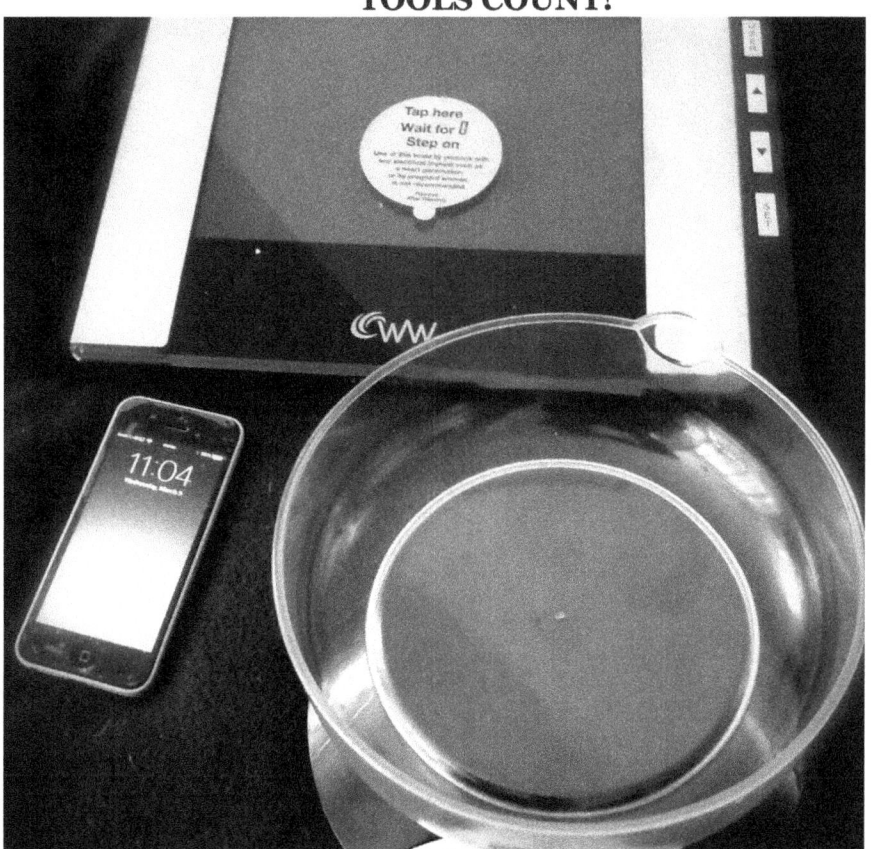

I can't stress enough how important it is to accurately track the food you eat. The Carb values for every meal, (including snacks), must be tracked and entered into the application for this plan to succeed.

Tools

To make my arsenal even stronger, I acquired a couple of must-have tools. These were the most important weapons I have. Without them, the plan is nearly impossible to manage.

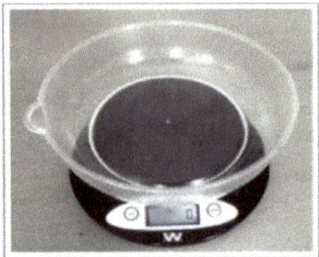

The first tool is a **kitchen scale** to precisely measure the portions I was consuming in my dishes.

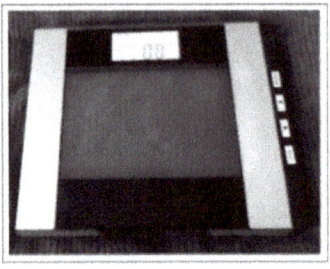

The second tool - what I call "the ultimate judge" - is a **bathroom scale**. I weigh myself every morning and get a realistic picture of my progress.

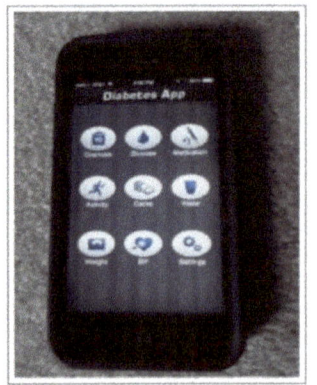

The App
Finding a way to keep precise track of all the key factors of the plan led me to an application that I could run on my Smartphone. In addition to tracking carbs, the app had the ability to track and display other key health areas, clearly and easily.

For my strategy, I figured out what key features in the app would be most useful for me, and which ones might become useful as I progressed towards my goal.

On the home screen of the app you see 9 buttons. You simply tap the one you want to activate.

50 Carbs

*The parts I used are **in boldface**.*

Overview: here you can see all the results according to the information you enter on one screen.

Settings: here is where you set the application to respond to the settings you enter for all the functions. For example I entered the limit of 50 carbs for my plan here.

Carbs: this one is the main key to the program. When activated, you have access to a vast database of food and their carb values. With more than 200,000 items, it sometimes got confusing to accurately enter the portions I was eating. It took me a few days to learn it.

Glucose: this one is very helpful for people with diabetes who want to keep track of their glucose levels. I perform the "out of bed pinch test" every morning. Tracking this in the app gives me peace of mind that my diabetes is under control.

Weight: I found this one to be the ultimate judge. The key is to weigh my body daily, and under the same conditions. I enter my weight in the morning, after the bathroom and before breakfast.

Blood Pressure: If you want to keep track of your blood pressure, enter here the info after you check it.

Medication: If you want to keep track of the medications you take here is the place to do it. I didn't find it useful in my case so I kept it blank.

Water: didn't see also any practical use of entering how many glasses I drink a day.

Activity: If you exercise here is where you enter your workout routine. Although I walk a couple of miles a day I found that light exercise alone to be irrelevant for losing weight. If you go deep and overdo it, your appetite could actually increase greatly.

Here's a quick example of how to use the Carb Feature...

When I open the carb section in my smartphone, a blue bar appears at the top. This line represents the 50 carb number I set.

As I cruise through the day, eating and entering my food choices, the blue bar starts changing to a green. Once I reach my pre-set carb limit, the green bar turns into a solid green bar. If I keep eating, the green bar starts turning red, indicating the extra carbs I'm eating.

I think is very important to deeply study all the functions of this section of the app. You need to become comfortable with easily and accurately entering the food you consume. The veracity of your results depends on the accuracy of these entries.

My App Choice

As an iPhone user, I went to the App Store and searched for applications that were targeted towards diabetes management. There are several very good apps - some free, some with a reasonable price tag.

I selected "The Diabetes App," which comes in two versions. From my experience, they both work well, with the "free" download giving me all the features I used for the 50 Carbs plan. Again, the main tracking features I look for are:

Glucose
Carbs
Weight

I also took a look at the Android store and found there were several apps that would do the job, though I did not personally use them.

If you like to share your updates, or see updates from other people who are managing their health, there are several popular applications that leverage social media/user group types of functionality.

You don't have to be diabetic to use these apps! The key is to track and react consistently, every meal, every day!

Chapter 9
The First Weeks

THE FIRST WEEK

The first week began with me investigating the carbs in the food that I regularly consumed. Using my app, I entered the information, including portion sizes as best I could.

SURVEY SAYS…

After analyzing the first couple of week's data, I was shocked to realize that I was consuming an average of 400 grams of carbs a day! How could that possibly be?

Let's take a look at what I was consuming in a typical day.

Breakfast: approx.130 carbs
- 3 scrambled eggs
- 3 slices of bacon
- salsa (4 spoons)
- 2 slices of sourdough bread
- butter/jelly
- sweet roll
- glass of orange juice
- 2 cups of coffee

Mid-day snack: approx. 75 carbs
- piece of pound cake
- butter and jelly
- cup of coffee

Lunch: approx. 150 carbs
- Hamburgers or sandwiches
- french fries

Afternoon snack: approx. 75 carbs
- chocolate chip cookie, or bowl of ice cream, or fruit

Dinner: - approx. 150 carbs
- salad
- pasta
- meatballs
  or
- pizza
- dinner roll

Before bed snack: approx. 50 carbs
- a bag of chips or a cookie

Well, that certainly wouldn't work! How can I trim all those carbs from my regular meals?

I noticed something very interesting. The spices and the techniques I used to cook my food had only a moderate impact in my carb daily allowance. I was able to bring out all of the flavors, turning every meal into a delicious treat!

One of my first goals was to try to find the perfect carb allowance number to put in the carb table. The number needed to reflect the level of hunger I could stand without feeling uncomfortably hungry.

I started by setting my daily carb allowance to 80.

I used a small kitchen scale as I prepared my meals. I entered the exact weight portions of the food, and the app calculated the carbs.

I found that at 80 carbs, my hunger levels were practically non-existent, and that my sugar glucose came down a little bit. A good start!

I then lowered my target to 70 carbs, and again – hunger was under control.

So… I dropped the number again, this time to 60 carbs. I was still feeling good, and still seeing good results.

Finally I reached the number of 50 carbs a day. I concluded that was the perfect number for me. The food intake would leave me a little bit hungry, but easily manageable, and nothing compared to the level of hunger you get by the third or four week of a diet.

This was something I could endure without major trauma.

My master plan was coming together. I was motivated; I had a few tools and good information.

I learned that if you want to keep your present weight you have to consume around 70 or 80 carbs a day. If you want to lose weight at a moderate pace you have to consume around 50 carbs a day, and if you want to go into the "crash" mode you have to stay around 30 carbs a day.

Chapter 10
Breakfast

MY NEW BREAKFAST

Here is where the carb negotiating started.

I began by identifying the key culprits that were running up the numbers. I went after the usual suspects - the 2 slices of sourdough bread, the jelly, the sweet roll and the orange juice. These bad boys accounted for about 99% of the total carb count of my breakfast.

I knew I could eat the 3 eggs, the bacon and the coffee "for free." The salsa would add 1 carb per spoon. It added enough enjoyment to the meal so I accepted the number and kept it in the lineup. I traded out the bread and jelly for low carb versions.

Here's what I changed.

Replaced the 2 slices of sourdough (60 carbs) with1 slice of multi-grain bread (13 carbs)

I spread butter and sugar-free jelly on top, and sprinkle a few little pieces of nuts like pecans, pine nuts or walnuts on it. Mmm... so delicious!

- Eliminated the sweet roll

- Eliminated the orange juice from my diet – I don't need it.

If I'm thirsty I drink a cold flavored tea (like Snapple Peach) or make myself a berry smoothie with no more than 6 carbs.

If I crave some kind of bread or wrapper to complement my eggs, bacon and salsa, I use one half of low carb tortilla (3 gr.). Sometimes one quarter will do. Sometimes I use only a quarter, or my new favorite bread - "lavash." It tastes good and there are some very low-carb versions.

This brings my breakfast to a total of 15 gr. to 20 gr. instead of 130 gr. and the end result is incredibly satisfying.

So this was the look of my new breakfast plate for a few weeks:

3 scrambled eggs with 3 slices of bacon, one slice of perfectly toasted multigrain bread with butter, sugar-free blueberry jelly and sprinkles of some kind of nuts. **I eat slowly and enjoy the taste of every bite.** This kind of meal lets me start the day with a full tank.

There are thousands of low carb breakfast options and many use a lower amount of carbs, but this kind of breakfast worked for me.

I've always really loved bread. As far as I know, multigrain bread is the best way I can get my regular daily slice of bread fix (and not overdo the carbs), without going to a true low-carb bread.

If I wanted to replace the multigrain bread with a low carb bread, my breakfast would be 4 carbs instead 15. One consideration is cost. A low-carb loaf is 3 times more expensive than a regular loaf of bread.

Here's a quick look at the changes I made to lower my morning carb intake while still enjoying a satisfying breakfast. Quite a difference in carbs, but still loaded with flavor. Check this out!

OLD BREAKFAST	NEW BREAKFAST
3 scrambled eggs	3 scrambled eggs
3 slices of bacon	3 slices of bacon
salsa (4 spoons)	salsa (1 spoon)
2 slices of sourdough bread	1/2 low carb tortilla
butter	butter
jelly	sugar-free blueberry jelly
Sweet roll	1 slice of toasted multi-grain bread
Orange juice	flavored tea
Coffee	Coffee
128 Carbs (approx.)	**15 – 20 Carbs (approx.)**

Pepe's Scrambled Eggs

On my quest to extract the maximum flavor of food for making a meal an enjoyable experience I've taken on the ageless classic breakfast – scrambled eggs with bacon and toast.

Here is my version of this satisfying and quick meal with only 2 carbs per serving. Add two more if you add salsa.

I find it to be important when you eat your meal that all the ingredients are done simultaneously. Sometimes while you wait for one of the ingredients to be done the others get cold and the experience gets a little bit diluted.

Breakfast

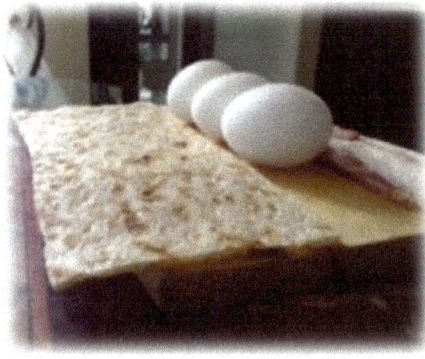

Ingredients

3 large eggs
2 slices of bacon
1 lavash portion
1 tbsp. vegetable oil
Salt and Pepper

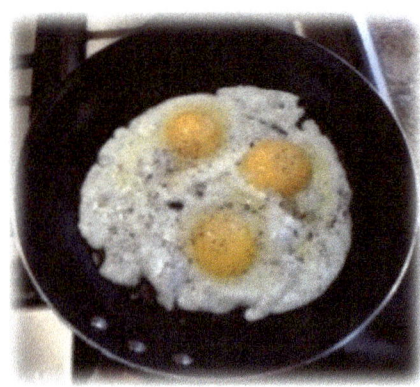

Heat the oil in a 12-inch non-stick pan. Once it is hot, crack the 3 eggs in the pan, just like you were going to make fried eggs. Add salt and pepper to taste. Let the white part get cooked, using your spatula to open the whites so they cook through without disturbing the yolks.

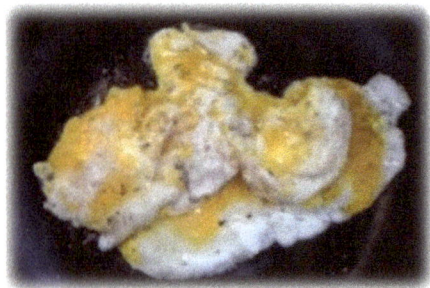

Once the whites look cooked, break the yolks and fold the eggs with your spatula a few times. Keep cooking until the yolks looks a little bit under cooked; not runny, not over cooked.

While the eggs are cooking, cook the bacon. Put the lavash in your toaster. If you like it crackling toasted (my favorite) let it run for one cycle or if you want it only warm pop it out of the toaster sooner.

50 Carbs

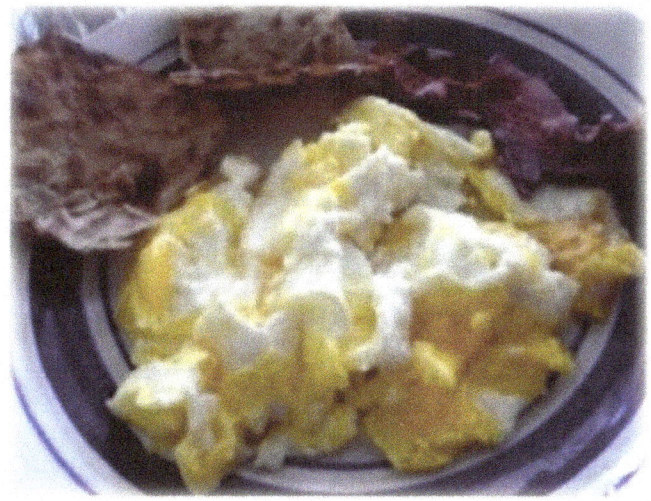

    This is to me the way to get the maximum flavor out of an egg, I find the white part to be flavorless but important for bonding. All the flavor is the yolk. I don't really like them runny, I think cooking the white part of the egg fully and then breaking the yolk and scrambling them enhances the flavor of scrambled eggs greatly.

Chapter 11

Snacks

MID MORNING AND MID AFTERNOON SNACK

"My name is José, and I love to snack."
There, I said it!

A few hours after breakfast and lunch, my body knocks and says "GIMME A SNACK!!!"

I used to calm my appetite with different treats - a piece of pound cake, a cookie, a bowl of ice cream or a large piece of fruit (oranges. pineapple, apples...). Sometimes I'd even make myself a sandwich. The snack was never the same, but one thing I know - I was consuming around 50 carbs in these "between" meals.

Sadly, most of the fruits that I love (mangoes, figs, pineapple, apples, grapes, bananas) are very high in carbs. A serving portion of 100 grams contains over 20 carbs.

Carb-friendly fruits include blackberries, melons, watermelons, peaches, strawberries and plums. A 100-gram serving contains under 10 gr.

I found a few options that would help me bring my "betweens" down from 50 carbs to 10 or less. If I was thinking about something sweet I'd enjoy a bowl of low carb ice cream, or grab a bowl and mix a few berries with some whipped cream from an aerosol can. If I was really motivated I'd build a delicious wrap by lightly frying half of a low carb tortilla in butter, then adding fresh blackberries or blueberry jelly and a few nuts sprinkled on top.

If I were feeling like something salty, I'd help myself to a serving of humus and a few stalks of celery. Other choices might be a piece of

50 Carbs

cheese, a small piece of chicken or a hard boil egg. I try not to go over 8 carbs.

JOSÉ'S GUACAMOLE

This is my most celebrated recipe. I don't know what it is that makes people react wildly. After the first bite they make a funny face, then break into a dance and a let out a loud "Mmmmm...." People really love it.

My guacamole is a great choice for snacking (believe it or not you can use pork rinds as chips if you want stay in the low carb mode). It's also a great side dish that can complement any kind of meat. Guacamole is a fresh, rich, healthy way to treat your body to a high quality fuel. A 4-ounce portion has about 4 carbs.

People keep asking me for the recipe. It is very simple to make – and this is the first time I'm going to reveal my masterpiece!

INGREDIENTS (3 portions)
1 large Haas avocado
1/4 of a yellow or white onion
1 large clove of garlic
one bunch of cilantro (if you can use only the leaves it will be better)
   the juice of 1 large lime
   1/4-cup virgin olive oil
   2 serrano peppers to start
   1/2 teaspoon of salt

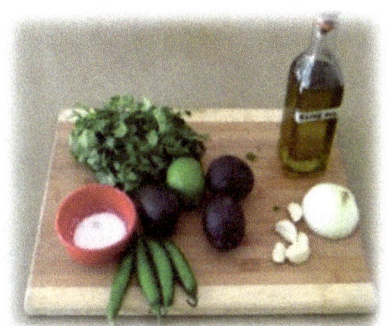

Theses portions are a good starting point. If you need more just increase the ingredients accordingly.

Put the avocado aside and chop all the other ingredients in your food processor until the texture gets to look like "pesto."

Snacks

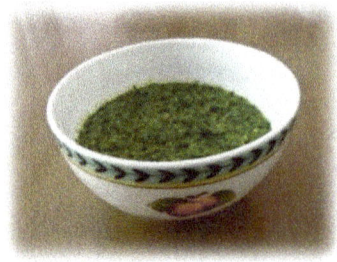

At this point you are going to taste it and determine if something is missing. If it's too dry you can add more olive oil. If it's not hot enough you can throw in another Serrano. Adding more lime can bring down the heat of the peppers or mellow out too much garlic.

If it needs more salt add more salt. You can keep mixing again and again in your food processor until the flavor is right.

You can make this guacamole "pesto" one day in advance. Just store it properly in your refrigerator.

When it's time to serve it, I cut the avocado into little pieces and fold them gently into the guacamole pesto. ENJOY!

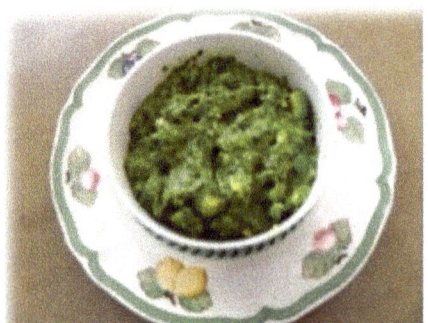
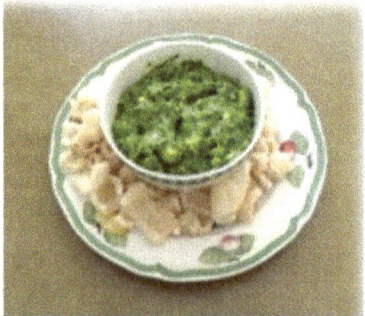

José's Guacamole. Add some pork rinds for a little crunch!

FLAXSEED BREADS

Bread… my favorite food choice when I'm hungry. There is something about it that, without it, my meals feel incomplete. I always feel the need to have a piece of bread or a tortilla to accompany my meals. Too bad they are fully loaded with carbs.

50 Carbs

I recently discovered Flaxseed Meal flour and its amazing properties. If you read the label info on the side of the package you'll see what I'm talking about. I use it to make my own delicious low carb bread. The carb value is practically zero, and the high fiber content per serving helps you to stay regular.

This recipe allows me to satisfy my bread love affair without breaking the carb meter.

Using the same ingredients I bake 3 different types of bread. The only thing that changes is the cooking tray.

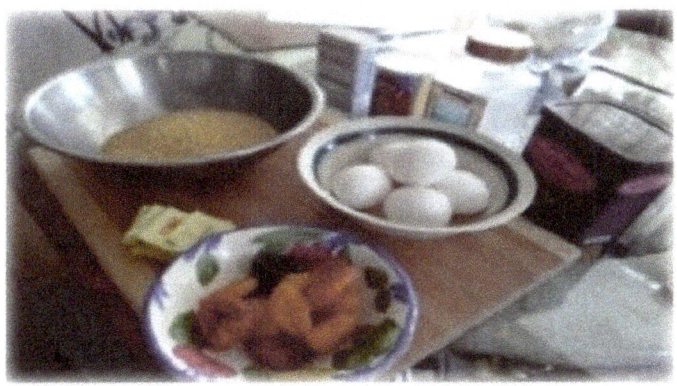

Ingredients

Flax seed meal	2 Cups
Baking Powder	1 Tbsp.
Salt	1 Tbsp.
Splenda	2 Tbsp.
Eggs	5 beaten
Vegetable oil	1/3 Cup
Water	1/2 Cup

The carb portion of the basic bread recipe using only the ingredients above is 1 gr. per serving. There is nothing too exiting about the flavor – it's decent for a sandwich or in a meal where the

Snacks

bread is not the star...until you spice it a little bit with some herbs.

Adding the following ingredients makes the serving around 6 gr. but turns the bread into a treat. Worth it for me.

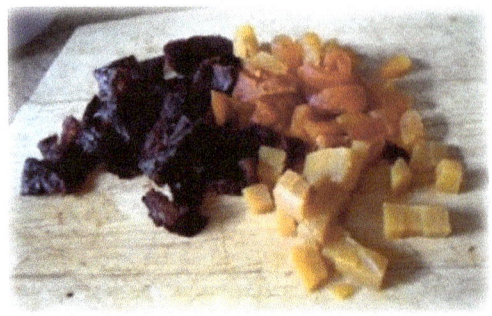

Dried Fruit	60 gr
Unsweetened Cocoa Powder	3 Tbsp.
Cinnamon	1 Tbsp.
Splenda	4 Tbsp. (total of 6)

Heat your oven to 350 degrees.

Put all the dry ingredients in a bowl. Mix them well with a spatula until they all are evenly blended.

Cut the dry fruit in little bite-sized pieces and sprinkle them one by one in the bowl. Avoid big clusters!

Add the oil, the water and the beaten eggs. Mix them gently but quickly with a spatula until everything is evenly blended, forming a wet dough.

You only have about a minute to mix the dough to keep it manageable.

Dump the mix into your cooking tray and put it in your 350 degrees oven for 25 to 30 minutes.

50 Carbs

If you want to add a chocolate frost to your breads I recommend this easy recipe.
8 ounces whipped cream cheese
6 Splenda packets
3 tbsp. of unsweetened cocoa powder

Whip all the ingredients (either by machine or by hand) until it's a uniform chocolate color. It is ready to be spread on any of these breads, and adds only 2 carbs per serving to the treat.

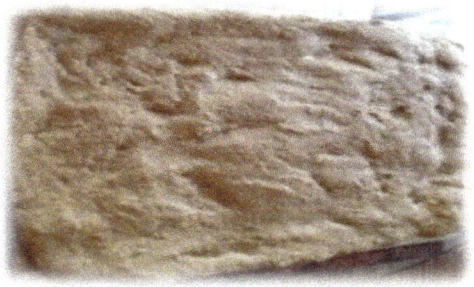

"Focaccia Type Bread" baked in 1/2 sheet tray. Great for sandwiches !

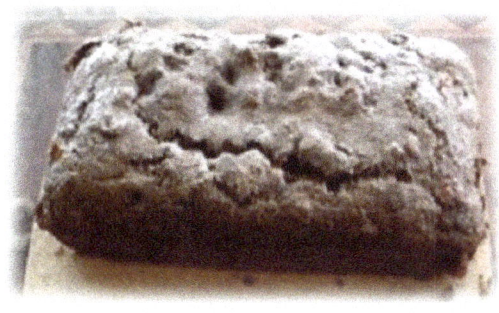

"Pound Cake Type Bread" baked in meatloaf or bread tray

"Cup Cakes" baked in a 12-cupcake tray

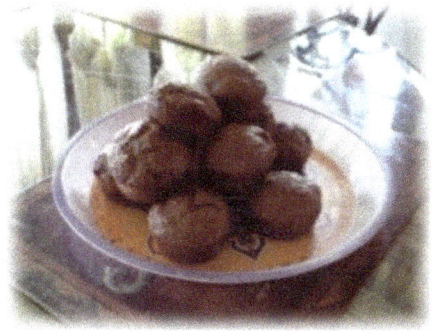

I love to cut these delightful cupcakes in half horizontally and pop them in the toaster for one cycle. I enjoy them every day with a good cup of coffee. Great for breakfast or mid-afternoon snack.

Snacks

AVOCADO GREEN SALSA
Ingredients

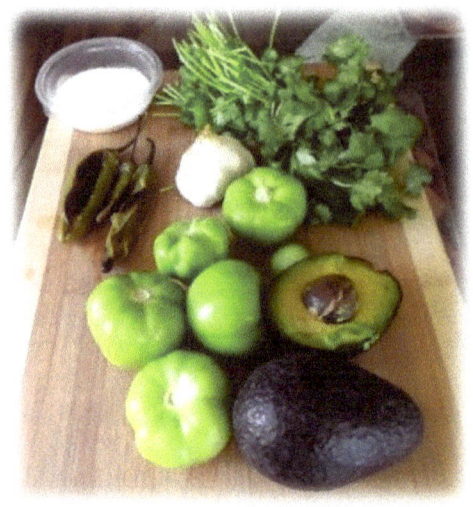

4 medium tomatillos, toasted, rinsed and roughly chopped
3 garlic cloves, peeled and roughly chopped
4 Serrano peppers, roasted and roughly chopped
About 1/4 cup (loosely packed) roughly chopped cilantro, thick lower stems cut off
1 large avocado pitted, flesh scooped from skin and roughly chopped
Salt to taste

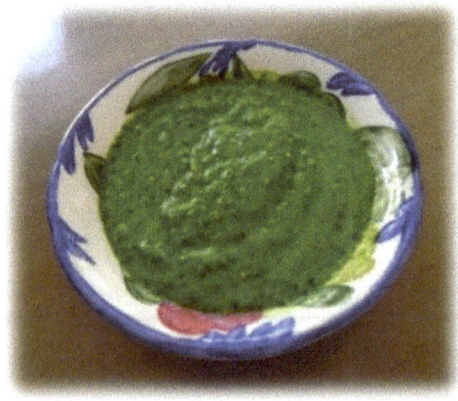

In a blender or food processor, combine the tomatillos, garlic, Serrano peppers, cilantro and 1/2 cup of water. Process to a coarse puree. Add the avocado and pulse until nearly smooth. Pour into a salsa dish. Taste and season with salt, usually about 1 teaspoon.

SALSA NEGRA
Ingredients

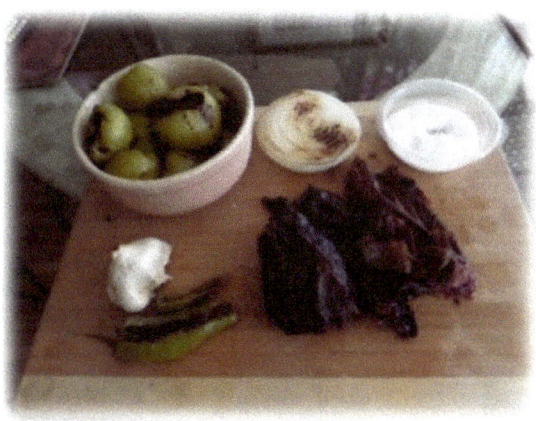

6 (medium) roasted tomatillos, roughly chopped

4 garlic cloves, peeled and roughly chopped

4 roasted pasilla peppers and 4 guajillo peppers rehydrated, roughly chopped

4 Serrano peppers roasted and roughly chopped

1/3 white onion

Salt

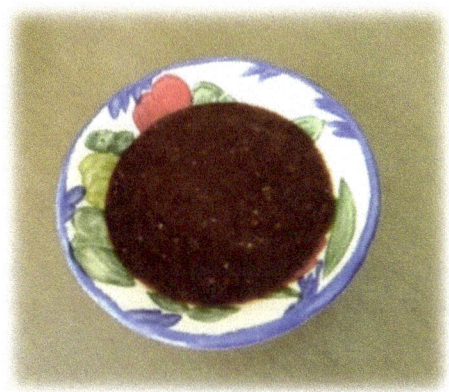

In a blender or food processor, combine the tomatillos, the Pasilla and Guajillo peppers, garlic, Serrano peppers and ½ cup water. Process to a coarse puree. pulse until nearly smooth. Pour into a salsa dish.. Taste and season with salt, usually about 1 teaspoon.

There are many low carb snack products in the market from cookies to muffins to chocolates - you name it. As I said earlier you have to be always prepared to kick HUNGER in the sprinkled nuts. If you can afford to stock your pantry with low carb products, go ahead and do it.

Chapter 12

Lunch and Dinner

LUNCH

Worst joke ever.
"Knock, knock."
"Who's there?"
"HUNGER , and I'm wearing a cup!"

About 5 hours after breakfast, my body was ready for another large meal. I'd usually make a run (ok, a drive) to a nearby hamburger joint that had all kinds of burgers and sandwiches on the menu.

My typical choice was a double burger, with a medium order of french fries, catsup and a chocolate or blueberry muffin. This combination would clock in at around 100 carbs. This would bring my running carb count to more than double my daily target, and I was only halfway through my day.

My New Lunch

I realized that in order to stay on target for a 50-carb day, lunch had to come in at around 10 carbs.

I could eat any kind of meat, (0 carbs), with an existing side dish like guacamole, or grilled vegetables, or a portion of humus (around 5 carbs). Adding half of a low carb tortilla (3 gr.), would bring my lunch down to around 10 grams of carbs instead 150.

Lunch and Dinner

I said farewell to my burger joint buddies and hello to my kitchen. I began to prepare my meals – lunch and dinner – in advance. I would make batches of deliciously satisfying soups and casseroles in 4 to 8 portion sizes. Every ingredient was carefully calculated to make each portion around 10 carbs. Preparing my food this way allowed me to have instant access to healthy, delicious meals.

Here's an example of an easy to prepare, easy to enjoy meal.

"chilaquiles negros" casserole (4 portions)
Ingredients

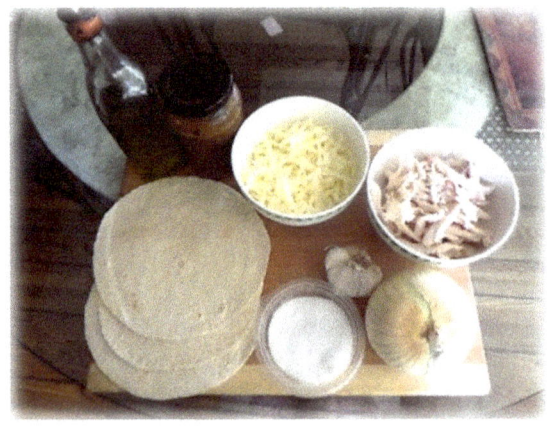

4 low carb tortillas cut in strips and fried
1 half of breast of shredded chicken, cooked
8 spoons of "dried peppers salsa"
mozzarella cheese

I prepare this like a lasagna.

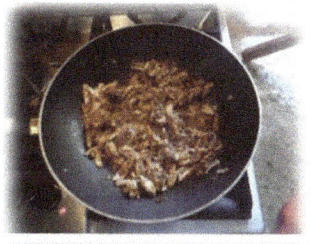

Place a layer of shredded chicken, dried peppers salsa, and mozzarella cheese on top of the tortilla.

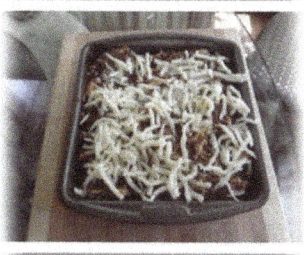

Build a second layer.
Bake it until the cheese melts.
Divide it into four equal portions.

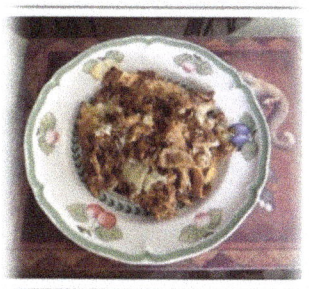

I eat one portion, and put the other three into the fridge. I now have three portions of awesomeness done and ready to eat whenever I need. I pop it into the microwave and reheat slowly (at 50% power).

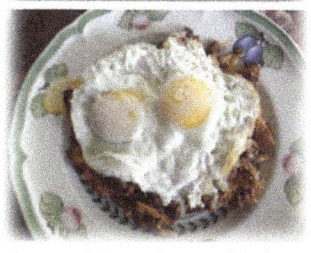

If I'm feeling a bit hungrier, I sometimes add a couple of fried eggs on top. This is still one of my favorite meals, and still around 10 carbs per serving.

Salad

How good is salad? A portion of a good spring salad loaded with tomato, red onions, feta cheese, apple, a few dry cranberries, radishes, red cabbage, and avocado drizzled with a bit of Ranch, Italian or Greek dressing will come in around 12 carbs.

Lunch and Dinner

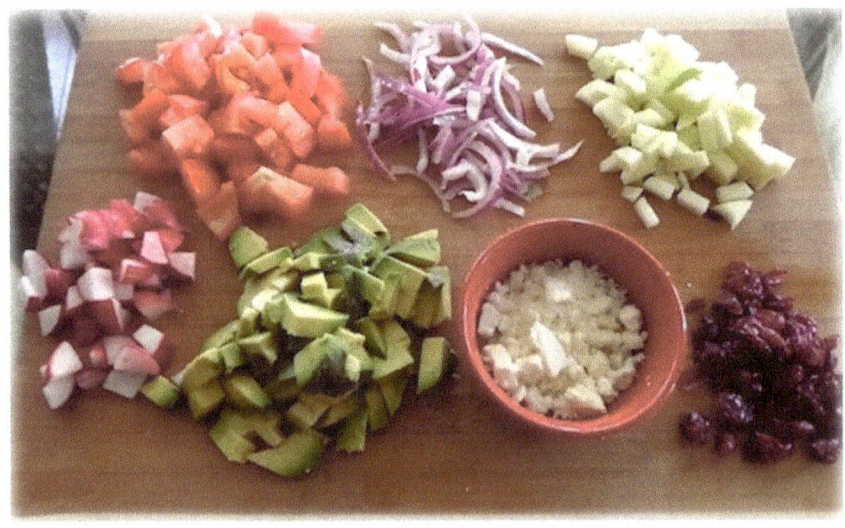

Now add some chicken, or about 4 oz. of sliced steak, or a can of tuna and you have a great meal. You will love it. Your body will love it. Happiness for lunch, or dinner!

Who doesn't love LASAGNA???

I think the word "Lasagna" must mean "yes, please" in some language. I love it so much that I had to keep it in my life. So I made a few changes and BOOM! - here it is! I substituted fresh slices of squash for the pasta, and every time I make it I say "Thanks, Amigo!"

SQUASH/MEAT LASAGNA RECIPE

Here's a nice a simple recipe that I cook very often. This delicious, carb-friendly dish is prepared in 4 or 8 serving batches, with only 6 gr. of carbs per serving, It stores well and is easy to reheat in the microwave for an instant meal.

Ingredients for an 8-serving tray

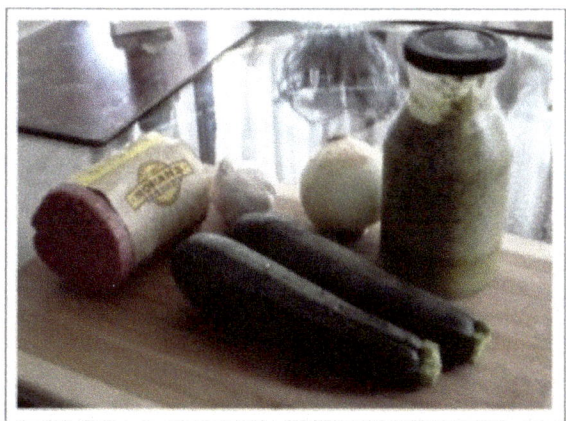

Ground Beef	2 pounds
Squash	4 fruits sliced
Yellow Onion	1 small
Garlic	4 large cloves
Salsa (green, red)	1 1/2 cups
Vegetable oil	4 Tbsp.
Monterey or mozzarella	8 ounces
Salt and pepper	To taste

Put the oil into a large frying pan to get medium hot.

Chop the onion and the garlic in small pieces and throw them in the hot pan and let them cook for a couple of minutes. The appetizing strong smell in the kitchen, just before they start getting brown lets me know that it's time to add the ground beef. I quickly separate the ground beef chunks into tiny pieces inside pan, add salt and pepper to taste, mix well all the ingredients and let them start cooking.

After a few minutes the beef releases all the juices that are loaded with flavor.

Continue cooking it for a couple of more minutes to let the juices reduce a little bit. Now it's time to add the salsa.

Lunch and Dinner

Let them cook all together for a few more minutes.

Before you turn it off, check for taste and add more spices if needed. Reach for a "not too wet thick texture" for spreading it as one of the lasagna two layers.

In the meantime cut the squash into thin long layers.

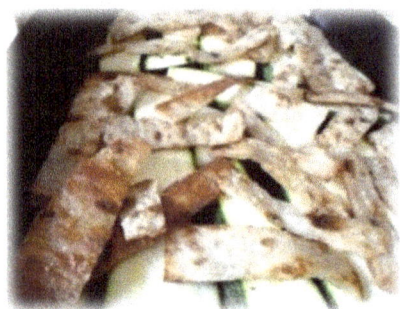

Before I started layering my 14" by 8" pan, I add a last minute improvisation. I add a few strips of a delicious lavash- a flat bread type I found in a local market. I fry them to add crunch and they become my fourth layer, at only 2 carbs per serving.

Set your oven temperature to 350 degrees - it's time to assemble the lasagna.

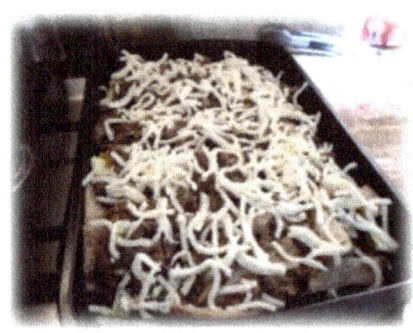

Divide all the ingredients in two parts.
Cover the bottom of the pan with the first 1/2 of the squash
Spread 1/2 of the lavash strips (optional)
Spread 1/2 of the meat ragù mixture
Sprinkle 1/2 of the Cheese

Repeat the layers again and put the tray in the 350-degree oven for 25 minutes.

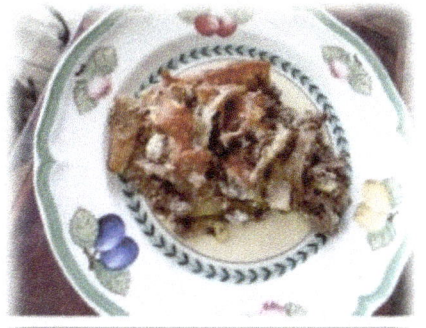

Serve

Once the food is cooked and has reached room temperature I cut the dish into 8 servings of 6 carbs each.

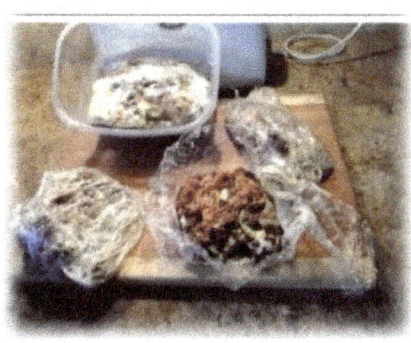

Storage

I wrap them individually in plastic paper and store them in a plastic tub in the refrigerator.

When I'm hungry I take one of this packages and heat it the microwave oven for 4 minutes at 50 % power.

Make the most of your cooking time

It helps a lot to make batches 4, 6 or 8 serving-sized casseroles, desserts, soups or vegetables in advance. When I have to eat and I don't have time to cook, my meal could be ready in 10 minutes. Most importantly, I feel protected, like these prepared portions are the bullets I need in my battle against HUNGER.

Chapter 13

Cookware

THE RIGHT TOOL FOR THE JOB

I strongly recommend using the appropriate kitchenware to cook your meals. It really greatly enhances the flavor of your food and makes the presentation aspect of your plates appetizing. These are some of the tools I use to cook my meals.

12-INCH STAINLESS PAN

My favorite pan for frying any kind of meat is a 12-inch stainless 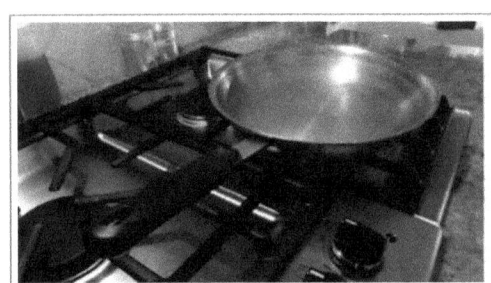 steel pan. I use it for everything from salmon, pork chops, chicken, steak, bacon and many more. I see a lot of chefs using the same type of pan in all kind of restaurants or on the cooking shows.

There's something about this vessel that makes food, and especially meat, release all the hidden flavors. It sears the food in a way that leaves an appetizing outer crust. After lifting the meat from the pan you can scrape the bottom with a liquid (wine, chicken broth) and there you have a delicious light sauce for your plate. All those delicious flavors go on your plate and nothing goes to waste. It makes you feel like you are having a plate coming from a fancy restaurant. At first some of the food might stick a little bit in the pan but after a few

50 Carbs

uses it develops a natural non-stick coating.

IMPORTANT REMINDER...

Remember to always allow enough time for the food to cook without rushing it, especially steaks. They don't like to be flipped over and over.

After spicing a steak with some kind of rub, I'll cook one side for about 4 minutes (depending on the thickness of the meat) for "rare" and 5 minutes for medium without disturbing it.

I flip it to the other side and cook for about a minute less than the first side (3 minutes for rare, 4 minutes for medium). Then I'll throw a few drops of wine in the pan and scrape the bottom, adding the flavors from the pan to the flavors of the wine for a great light sauce that takes the experience up a step. This is a great treat, with no additional carbs.

UP NEXT - THE DOUBLE GRIDDLE !

My next favorite pan is a double griddle. Before I discovered the stainless steel pan this one was my "work horse."

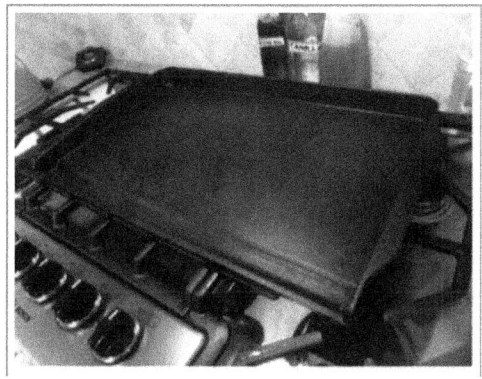

I love the fact that I can cook 2 items at the same time on this griddle. I place it on top of two of the burners in my stove. It fits perfectly and gives me the option to control the heat of each side independently. This is the only type of pan I know that gives me similar textures and flavors to those of the professional griddles in restaurants at home.

I can cook my steak on one side and cook stuff like onions, peppers or potatoes on the other side. It's great for breakfast, too. I can cook eggs, pancakes, bacon, even quesadillas at the same time.

I love to make "sweaty tortillas" this way. I prepare some steak with my favorite spices, then cut it into little taco-sized pieces and throw it on the griddle. On the other side of the grill I put some chopped veggies – peppers, onions – and grill them up. After a couple of minutes I throw a couple of tortillas to cover the meat while it finishes cooking. Then I take the tortillas and I mop up some of the meat juices.

I put the "sweaty tortillas' on a plate, add some of the meat and veggies, add a spoon of my guacamole or my salsa... wow!!.. I cannot tell you how wonderful and intense is this dish's flavor.

I go to heaven every time I eat this simple treat.

This meal would usually land at about around 70 carbs per serving. Under the 50 Carbs plan I use a low carb tortilla (or a half if I want to fill the "carb jar"). I do everything else as described above, and come in under 10 carbs per serving.

This is lunch or dinner for me some times, and believe me – I do not mind at all!

SAY "HELLO" TO THE MIGHTY DUTCH OVEN

There is no better method to cook food slowly than doing it with

50 Carbs

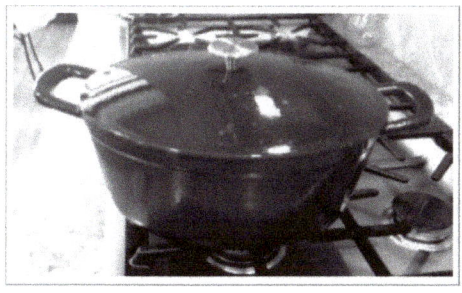

this pot. Things like chicken and other soups, sauces, and stews are just a few of many dishes that come out tasting delicious. The lid of this heavy pot really seals the vessel tight, not allowing any of the flavors to escape. Everything stays inside, where it belongs!

My chicken soup recipe (6 portions)

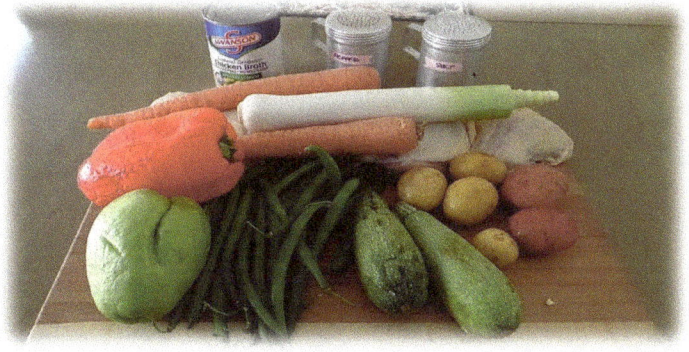

Ingredients:

6 chicken pieces (better with bones and skin)
1 finely chopped leek
2 carrots chopped
2 celery stalks chopped
1 bunch of green beans
1 red pepper chopped
2 cups of chicken broth or stock

Feel free to add more vegetables like potatoes, chayote, squash, corn, chickpeas if you want.

Cookware

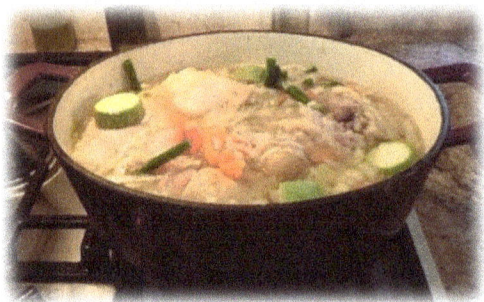

Put everything in the pot, bring it to a boil then reduce the fire to a simmer and cook for at least 1 hour.

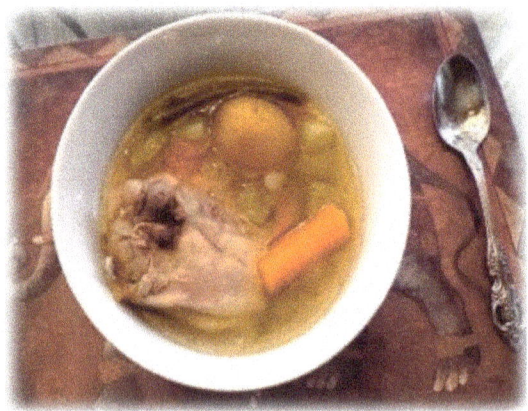

That's it! Hot and deliciously ready, perfect for those cold days.

According to my calculations, a large serving of soup with a leg and a thigh or a breast and lots of broth and vegetables has approximately 10 grams of carbs.

PEPPER STEAK

Here's another family favorite, perfectly designed for the Mighty Dutch Oven.

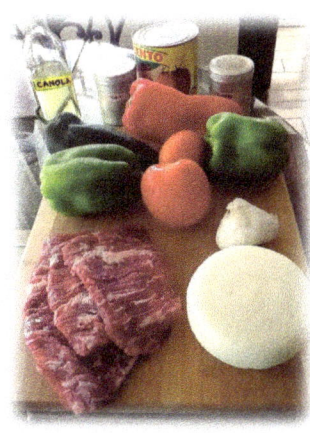

Ingredients:

1-pound steak cut into bite size strips

1/2 yellow onion chopped small

4 garlic cloves chopped small

1 green pepper cut into small strips

4 serrano peppers chopped into small pieces

1 can of tomato sauce

2 plum tomatoes without skin (optional)

Salt and pepper to taste

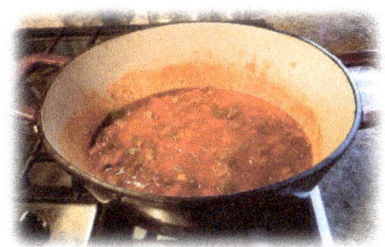

Start with the onions. Fry them for a couple of minutes. Add the garlic and cook for another couple of minutes. Then add the peppers, keep cooking for a few more minutes. Now, add the steak, cooking until the steak has released all the juices. Add the tomato sauce and tomatoes. Bring to a boil and then simmer for at least 1 hour.

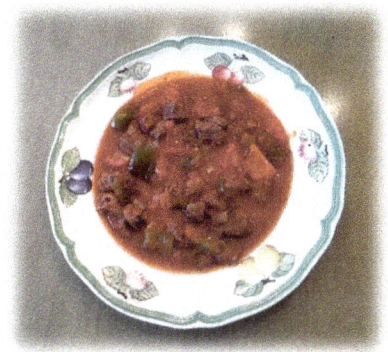

Serve with passion!

Chapter 14
Out and About

WHEN IN ROME…

The old saying "A man's home is his castle" may have been ok way back when, but I know a whole lot of women who'd say "no way José!" I'm changing it up a bit, and going with "This man's kitchen is his fort!" Give it time – it will catch on!

I have control over what goes on, in and out of my fort. But what happens when I venture out into other lands, where the forts are different and the food prepared differently? Parties, restaurants, family gatherings, music festivals, even a trip to the mall can have hidden traps and temptations aimed at pulling me away from my 50 carb vocation.

No doubt, my will power gets tested.

I follow some basic, sensible practices to stay true to my plan. I have to remember to stay away from bread, heavy sauces, pasta, pizza, rice, beans, tortillas, potatoes, sweet drinks, cakes, and some fruits. Just one serving of one of these products can chew up a whole day's worth of my carb allowance.

When I'm eating in a restaurant I can quickly assemble a decent meal for around 20 carbs. Not bad when you are out of your domain. I look through the menu for baked or grilled meats. I'll add a side of vegetables like broccoli, and add a few dashes of Tabasco or 2 spoons of salsa if is available.

To make sure that I was not going to feel deprived, I sometimes carry with me an 8- inch square of lavash (a middle eastern bread) folded in a small plastic bag. It looks and tastes like a square flour tortilla, and adds a nice compliment to my meal, while adding only 4 carbs.

Occasionally if I'm eating a steak I'll order a baked potato, with salt, pepper and butter and eat only one half (14 carbs). Many times I only eat one quarter (7 carbs)

For desert I look for a fruit plate with berries and whipped cream (5 grams).

So – a hearty, flavorful meal that can clock in at around 20 carbs. No suffering here!

Sometimes I'm confronted with a sandwich or a hamburger as my only option. No problem. I'll break it all down and rebuild the meal. First I separate all the meat from the bread. Then, I clean the bread and cut it in half. I discard one half and re-assemble the sandwich again using the remaining half. All the meat goes back in the remaining bread. I put back "un poquito" of the filler; I choose the low carb vegetables like lettuce, peppers, and avocados (the filler). A touch of olive oil and a dash of Tabasco keep it exciting. Before you know it, you have a pretty nice sandwich! If I can do the same with only one quarter of the bread - even better - it saves me at least 8 carbs.

This could cut my sandwich carbs from 50 carbs to a half or a quarter of that total. I walk out of the establishment feeling like I had a hamburger... it does the trick for me.

I specifically build this type of food based on my own lifestyle and what I'm used to eating. I think anybody can do the same and build a menu with food they are used to eating. Just enter the food you eat in your phone app. Look at the carb number. Is it too high? Use a smaller portion, find a substitute or eliminate it from your menu.

Here are a few additional tips I found during my own search for ways to deal with eating out.

- Can you get a sense of what the restaurant offers before you go?
- Check online – many places post their menus on their website, along with some information about off-menu options for different types of dining needs.
- Look for places that serve a la carte meals. This can help you mix and match foods that fit into your 50 Carb plan.
- Let your server know you're following a low-carb plan. Restaurants want their customers to have a great experience, and will often make suggestions and substitutions based on your needs. This may not always happen, especially in crowded casual restaurants, but go ahead and have the conversation.
- Simply prepared beats heavily sauced or breaded.
- Avoid deep-fried anything.
- Fresh vegetables instead of fries.
- Salads can be turned into satisfying meals when you add some meat or chicken.
- Have an omelet, filled with fresh low carb vegetables like spinach or mushrooms.

Put the breadbasket on someone else's table!

Remember - the goal is to build a menu of 50 carbs-a-day meals with all of the food ingredients you selected for your personal program. I found it to be a lot less stressful to have an idea of what I could eat during the day. I just shuffle my meal options and make every day a little different.

Chapter 15
Quick Notes...

FLAVOR FLAVOR FLAVOR

I've noticed something interesting when I eat the same meal but it is prepared differently. One version is prepared fairly plainly (read – dull!) and the other prepared with some spark (read – delicious). The plainer dish often leaves me hungry, and my body demands more food sooner.

The same dish with the flavor tweaked up using spices and seasonings that add little or no carbs makes the meal much more enjoyable, and keeps my body happier for a longer time.

I find myself using the basics like salt and pepper, and zesty additions like cumin to add a bit of sizzle. Nothing beats a good old onion, a zippy serrano pepper, and garlic is a must for most of my meals. Dried peppers, red pepper flakes, and oregano make the short list. I also make a nice dry rub for meats. Chile pasilla and chile guajillo add a nice smoky flavor to any meal.

For a sweeter twist, I take a bit of artificial sweetener, add a few drops of sugar-free coconut syrup, and drizzle it on top of fruits like cantaloupe, strawberries and nectarines. Any fruit that is not quite sweet or ripe enough will go from good to great!

SIMPLE MATH

My strategy called for consuming only 50 carbs a day. It was essential for me to get familiar with the "Diabetes App" so I could find the easiest and quickest way to enter the content of my meals accurately. Entering the correct food portions for each meal is the winning ticket.

To get better meals while staying within the 50 carbs a day budget, I learned how to divide portions so I could enter the correct numbers.

For instance if I wanted to add apple to a salad and used only one slice of apple, I'd enter only one slice to the carb count of the salad - not the whole apple.

I feel that a good one-portion salad can be built with 12 carbs. If you add 3.5 ounces of any kind of meat to the same salad you have a healthy, delicious meal that doesn't add any carbs.

BE PREPARED

I find it's very important to always be prepared with smart food you can readily eat.

When I get caught feeling hungry without my special food, the fight usually gets a lot tougher.

The best way I can describe the situation is like having no ammunition for the weapon you are using to fight your enemy, HUNGER. Suddenly, there it is, and you and your willpower have a real battle on your hands!

I often cook batches of 2, 4 or more servings/portions of foods like chicken soup, casseroles, meat dishes, and deserts that can be safely stored in my refrigerator, ready to reheat and serve at any time. The beauty of this is that I always have delicious food, with a carb value under 10 per serving, ready to go. This definitely gives you a lot of security; it's like having the perfect weapon within reach when your enemy – HUNGER – shows up!

CARB COINS

I've learned to ask myself every time I eat – "do you really need to eat the whole portion that's in front of you?" I challenge myself to leave some of the portion on the plate. Many times a half of a portion would be enough to satisfy me, and save me half the carbs of that particular item. Whatever you leave on the plate counts in your favor, and the more you lower the carbs the faster the weight disappears.

I compare this exercise to when I put the coins I'm carrying in my pocket into a jar. Before I know it, the jar is full of coins – over $100.00 that I can spend any way I want.

This jar full of "unspent carbs" is put towards losing weight more quickly. Believe me, it's a fun exercise!

You don't have to use the whole day's carb allowance. If you feel satisfied – then you're satisfied!

Chapter 16

Prepare For Takeoff

GET READY

Before you take off on your 50 Carb program, remember the concept; you are going to give your body the focus and quality time it needs to get back into shape. If you make it a priority you will be very happy with the results.

Think of a pilot getting ready for a long trip. Before his plane takes off he must have a destination and a flight plan to easily reach that destination. He knows that he's going to make a few stops to refuel. Before he jumps in the plane he inspects the outside, checks all the instruments in the panel and makes sure he has a survival kit in case of an emergency. He is prepared.

So, let's do our own pre-flight check.

Destination

Find out what the goal is for your first stop. Using the height/weight table, find the target range of weight and set your sights on reaching the upper number. Figure out how much weight you need to lose to get there. That is your first destination.

Height and Weight Chart by Gender

The following chart represents target weight ranges according to your height and frame size. It's broken out by gender - women to the

Prepare for Takeoff

left, men to the right.

WOMEN				MEN			
Height	Frame Size			Height	FrameSize		
Ft. In.	Small	Medium	Large	Ft. In.	Small	Medium	Large
4'10"	102-111	109-121	118-131	5'2"	128-134	131-141	138-150
4'11"	103-113	111-123	120-134	5'3"	130-136	133-143	140-153
5'0"	104-115	113-126	122-137	5'4"	132-138	135-145	142-156
5'1"	106-118	115-129	125-140	5'5"	134-140	137-148	144-160
5'2	108-121	118-132	128-134	5'6"	136-142	139-151	146-164
5'3"	111-124	121-135	131-147	5'7"	138-145	142-154	149-168
5'4"	114-127	124-138	134-151	5'8"	140-148	145-157	152-176
5'5	117-130	127-141	137-155	5'9"	142-151	156-160	155-176
5'6"	120-133	130-144	140-159	5'10"	144-154	151-163	158-180
5'7"	123-136	133-144	143-163	5'11	146-157	154-166	161-184
5"8	126-139	135-150	146-167	6'0"	149-160	157-170	164-188
5'9"	129-142	139-153	149-170	6'1	152-164	160-174	168-192
5'10"	132-145	142-156	152-173	6'2"	155-168	165-178	172-197
5'11"	135-148	145-159	155-176	6'3"	158-172	167-182	176-202
6'0	138-151	148-162	158-176	6'4"	162-176	171-187	181-207

Here's how I approached it. I am 5'9". The tables say that if you have a small frame, your weight should be between 142 and 151 pounds. For a medium frame, the range is 156 – 160 pounds. A large frame has a range of 155 – 176 pounds.

When I started I was 210 pounds, so I set my first goal at 176 – a loss of 34 pounds.

Second Stop

Since I reached my first goal fairly quickly and easily, I decided to keep going. Why not? I had a system and I figured out what worked for me. I found a lot of great recipes and came up with a bunch of my own. So – next stop, 160!

Final Destination

I was now in the zone, loving my new body, enjoying the new freedoms, enjoying new taste treats, loving the new energy sense of accomplishment. I kept true to the plan, and I've settled at a comfortable weight at the lower end of the scale.

Checking The Instruments

Smartphone app - set up, reviewed and understood. This means you:

- Know what each screen does
- Know how to enter the required information
- Know what the information means
- Know what to do with the information

Bathroom scale - in place and ready to use every morning. Routine set.

- Wake up
- Go to the bathroom
- Weigh yourself on the scale

I think a consistent routine is important. You'll get the most accurate results and have the best reading on your weight fluctuations. Every morning I weigh myself and enter the info into the app right away. I often take pictures of the scale's screen as a reminder, or as encouragement!

Kitchen scale - Operation understood, the display is clear and easy to read. Ready to use every time you cook.

This tool is very helpful in accurately measuring the right amount and weight of the ingredients I use in my recipes. It is also a great tool to help keep track of everything – especially the carbs - when you make large portions.

Cooking vessels - I care very much about extracting all the possible flavor a product renders. The right vessel and method of cooking is important. It will improve the whole experience. The finished presentation of the food you'll eat is part of that positive experience, just like when you're served a meal in first class.

Fuel - The most important element. Without it you cannot go anywhere. At this point you've done your research and have a basic idea of the food you are going to eat during the trip. You have a menu of some dishes that you can prepare and enjoy on your journey.

Prep early, Pack Smartly

Put aside a few hours one day a week in your calendar to prepare your carb conscious food batches. Make them delicious! Refrigerate them properly, and wrap them so you can eat them at home, or put them in your lunchbox if you're going to be out and about. You can make all kinds of dishes in advance; stuff like meatloaf, casseroles, breads, stews, hard-boiled eggs…. There are thousands of recipes on line - the choices are infinite.

These actions could be the ticket to a smooth weight reduction ride.

Once you fully understand how this whole plan works you will be able to open and close the gate that controls your weight. Having this ability at your command is an awesome power.

This is possible by simply analyzing every day the data you enter in your app. If all the numbers look okay- great! If you see that your weight went up that day, look at what you ate the day before. You can quickly identify what's causing the increase. Maybe the portions are too big, so next time use less or substitute ingredients to bring down the carbs.

Carbs and Calories - reminder.

I was very curious about why some days my weight fell faster than others. I noticed that on the days I was able to keep the carbs under 50 and the calories under 1000, my weight dropped faster. it seems like my body was responding to a carb diet and a calorie diet simultaneously.

We know that we can eat as much steak and bacon as we want, and the carb value would be zero. However, the calorie count goes through the roof! Use your common sense!

Chapter 17
Short Cuts

SHORT CUTS

When I first started this amazing program I wasted many days trying to make sense of what the heck was going on with my body. The weight was falling off at an incredible pace but it took me a few days to decode and analyze all the information. Once I understood the rhythm it was easy to ride along.

My body responded so well to this diet that it was beyond belief. My weight was dropping at a rate way faster than I was expecting. The way I prepared my carb-conscious food was 100% deliciously satisfying and made it easy to stay on the program. I kept asking my self "where is the catch?" So far I haven't found it. I don't know if you find it annoying to hear people coming up to you all day long with flattering comments. I have no problem with that!

I can't tell you how amazed I am to see how simple it is to open and close my personal "weight gate." It does not require any overwhelming amount of effort or food depravation from me. OK, I can tell you; I am very, very amazed.

I hope your journey will be like mine. I grew very comfortable with this new lifestyle, so much that I'm still on the program. I'm planning to adopt it for my lifetime. I still keep daily records of my meals and weight so I can tell my position. So far so good. I've been able to maintain my weight at 140 pounds for the last 6 months with no complaints.

As I began to master the running of the program, the first thing I started to pay close attention to was the kind of carb-acceptable foods my body enjoyed the most. I adapted my cooking around them. There were plenty of food options that I enjoyed. I'm aware that I have not even scratched the surface of the thousands of available foods that could fit inside the 50-carb boundaries. Just find the ones you like, get creative, adapt your meals around them, and prepare your own carb-controlled masterpieces.

I knew right away that if I could include all this good food in my diet in a smart and orderly way, my stomach would be almost satisfied and my body could stay under this program for long periods of time. What I mean by "almost satisfied" is managing the unavoidable state of hunger that all dieters have to face in order to make the pounds disappear. It can become stronger especially when you are reaching for the lower numbers for your frame. But it can be managed!

WHAT WORKED

The two most important requirements that made "The 50 Carbs Program" work for me were ***Commitment and Discipline***.

Commitment: I believe that the only way to succeed in any endeavor in life is to make a serious commitment to the task. If you can prove to your universe that you are prepared to endure any sacrifices that cross your path, for as long as is necessary until you reach your goal, eventually you'll succeed. That's the kind of commitment I made to my body.

Discipline: To me it's a combination of focus and determination. Here are the keys to the plan that required my discipline.

Count Everything

Do not skip entering the data of *everything* eaten during the day - *every day*.

If I could not enter it at the moment, I would enter it later in the day. Only by entering the information as accurately as possible would I know where I was standing. At first I didn't alter any of the products or portions sizes that I consumed. It didn't matter how bad it was - until I realized that I was cheating myself.

Be Organized

Being organized was very important. Besides entering the food I found it helpful to also input the right type of meal I was having (breakfast, dinner, snacks, or others).

Be smart and be prepared - not only with your own carb-friendly food but also with information about where the enemy is hiding. Use the good information within your smartphone app to help you win the day's battle.

Timing

I tried not to eat anything after 7 PM.

Analyze and Understand

Using the carbs section of the app I analyzed the results of every meal I had as the day progressed. This helped me manage the carb allowance for my next meal.

Create a Routine

I weighed my self every morning after the bathroom, wearing only my briefs. Registering my weight under the same daily conditions gave me a consistent and realistic way to detect even the smallest weight fluctuations, so I could deal with it accordingly.

Make Adjustments

Usually when your weight is not moving after a week something is wrong in your diet. Checking your food data from the previous couple of days makes it easy to find the culprit.

Calories

Some foods don't show a lot of carbs, but the calorie content is high. Watch for those days that exceeded 1500 calories. Too many calories in your diet could slow down or pause your progress. The ideal day for me was when I could keep my carbs under 50 and the calories under 1000. It's like having two faucets open at the same time.

Getting Close…

As with any diet the last few pounds are harder to get rid of and the weight drop occurs at a slower pace. If you are patient and you are comfortable during the ride I'm pretty sure you can continue your journey down until you say "stop."

In my case I decided to stop when I reached 137 pounds. I was starting to look too skinny, and if I went any lower I would be looking anorexic. Now I'm trying to maintain a weight that ranges between 140 and 144 pounds. Due to my height (5'9") I'm a few pounds below the lower range of the small frame. I like the way my body looks and feels, 100% diabetes free.

Keeping Score

This program is really like a game that involves your physical participation every day. Your goal is to check the scorecard – in this case your bathroom scale – every morning. It's pretty easy to tell how you did. Win, lose or draw – you lost a little weight, you gained a little weight, or you stayed the same. The more you finish your day below 50 carbs the more points you score. The reward is a faster weight drop. It's like stepping into the gas pedal to get to your destination quicker.

Your day is mined with food traps and temptation, so your will power is constantly tested. If you pass beyond the 50 carbs boundaries you lose the day's game, but if you stay inside the boundaries you win the day's game.

Celebrate Each Win

I can't help feeling victorious every time I "win." It's a high moment when the bathroom scale is displaying the score in your favor. It's like scoring a goal, or making a touchdown. Savor the moment, celebrate it, take a picture, find it inspiring and draw from it the strength you need to take you to the next challenge.

Handle the Bumps

When my weight goes up instead of down, I don't panic. One bad day is a manageable setback. To recover, the first thing I do is analyze the data from the day(s) before and find the foods that are causing the spike. I come up with a strategy to remedy the problem, execute it immediately, and look for the results the next day. I continue tweaking the strategy until I reach the desire result. I find the challenge entertaining!

Chapter 18

Go Get It!

There are thousands of diets on the market. Lots of them work well, though some of the programs can get very expensive and hard to maintain. Others require you to buy products from the sellers; others are very extreme. At the end of the day the real challenge for everybody is keeping the weight down for a long period of time - or for a lifetime.

From my own experience, the loss of weight is only temporary; you put in the work to bring your weight down to your goal. Then comes the next stage - perhaps the hardest - and that is keeping your weight down.

This is the biggest challenge all dieters face and where most of them fail. It seems to me that that during this cycle my body demands more fuel to keep it going and oh boy!! It really lets me know it.

I dropped most of the weight in the first 3 months and I have spent the last 6 months keeping my weigh stabilized at around 140 pounds.

It has not being an easy task. Hunger puts up a fight to the death against my will power and tries desperately to get me to give up.

I have been able to keep my weight around 140 pounds for 6 months already without suffering the punishment of the severe hunger. Otherwise it would have turned into a disaster.

I've had a few days where I've experienced constant hunger all day long. Thanks mainly to the food I prepare in advance along with the carb-friendly food in my pantry I have sensible food near me at all times.

So far I have been able to keep on the winning side in the fight against sharp hunger. I'm pretty sure that without my food my willpower would have surrendered to hunger a long time ago.

This period in the program has brought me some interesting observations.

To maintain my body in the 140-pound area I have to give my body the amount of food that a 140-pound body requires. For me this pretty much means eating the same food I was eating during the diet period. I'm adding a little more fruits and vegetables to my meals, but only a little.

The few times that I've eaten a portion heavy in carbs - stuff like regular bread, a piece of cake, candy, crumb- coated chicken, a full baked potato, and some fruits and vegetables with my meals, my weight went up between 2 to 3 pounds a week.

The bathroom scale lets me know pretty much the next day. By just coming back to the 50 Carbs program, I get back to my target weight in a few days.

I think it's okay to detour occasionally, but only for a very short period. Otherwise you will pay the consequences.

What makes this diet different from the others is that it focuses on eating good-tasting meals, designed and prepared by you under the 50 Carbs boundaries, using products easily available in any market. It works in the weight-loss phase, and it works as you maintain your loss.

The features of this diet let me build the ideal program to endure, in a kinder way, what in the past had been an ugly ride. It still takes focus and work but I will look great – slim and fit – for a long time. Believe me, it's worth it!!!

If you decide to try the 50 Carbs program, be patient. Don't get discouraged if you don't get results right away. Your body needs a few days to adapt to a new way of eating and to get familiar with and understand the new process.

It is important to make enough time in your schedule at least once a week, to prepare your food. How much ammunition do you need to endure the battle against hunger? That's up to you.

Don't freak out if after a couple of weeks into the program, for a few days, your body emits a peculiar scent. This is called ketosis and is the result of your body burning fat. It is fairly common in many low-carb diets. It's an indication that the carb-burning machine is in motion and working. It's a positive point to reach in the 50 Carbs diet.

Use your App. Remember you have 24/7 access to key carb, calorie and weight information. Look at it as often as you need to give you a perspective on how your day is going. Use that information to help you deal with it accordingly.

As far as I'm concerned, this 50 Carbs program worked incredibly well for me. It rid me of more than 60 pounds - making my appearance way more attractive - but most importantly made me "Diabetes Free." It also repaired other important factors related to my health such as high

blood pressure and high cholesterol. I keep hearing from a couple of doctors that this action added to my life at least 10 more years. I'll take it.

Chapter 19
One Year Later

APRIL 2015 - ONE YEAR LATER

One year has passed since I reached two of the most incredible achievements of my life - getting rid of my diabetes and losing over 60 pounds in only four months.

I feel it is very important to pass along my own experience during this year. Based on my previous attempts at dieting I expected this period would be the hardest, but with 50 carbs it was definitely survivable! This chapter should give you a realistic perspective of what to expect and what is involved to successfully run this amazing and effective program. I'll also share some strategies on following the 50 Carb plan without a smartphone application.

I can testify that the diet period is only a temporary sacrifice. If you are highly motivated you will most likely achieve your desired goal. It was a very positive experience for me. I was fully motivated and my will power was charged to the top. Watching my weight drop 5 pounds a week was amazing and inspiring. I did not want to stop, but once I did I realized I needed to make some adjustments.

A year ago I got so thin that I started to look almost anorexic. It took me a couple of months to gain 5 pounds, and that is where I determined I felt and looked the best. I've decided to hold on to it as long as I can.

To get to this point I had to go through the discipline of monitoring the diet through the app on my smartphone. I learned by heart the carb value and portion size of the few main items I use when I'm cooking and how my body was responding. I had entered every ingredient I used to build my meals every time - around 1000 times. I also weighed my self every morning and pinched my finger for a glucose test.

It was fascinating for me to be able to witness the dynamics of this process. I was able to detect and sometimes predict the smallest weight fluctuations. It was very helpful and encouraging to be informed by immediate access to key information.

Today I'm still under the 50 Carbs program boundaries. I'm not doing everything with as much discipline as I was in the beginning. I've developed routines that let me follow the plan by memory. Now I check my blood sugar once a week, weight my self every couple of weeks and I don't log my food intake on my smartphone. At this point it is unnecessary to keep doing that. The daily routine is pretty much the same. I have memorized the carb value and portion sizes of the few items that I use the most when I'm cooking. Keeping track of the accounting of 50 carbs a day is not a hard task. So far my numbers still look good.

Soon after this period began, the motivation and willpower that kept me going strong had wound down a lot, and the ugly face of constant hunger showed up. The fight to maintain my new weight became a steady issue. My body keeps clamoring for food all day long, as if it's trying very hard to get back the weight it once had. The "honeymoon" is over. I have always found this period of time to be the hardest challenge for any diet.

I feel very lucky to have discovered through the 50 Carbs method how to keep my body constantly fed, easing this misery without jeopardizing the goal achieved. So far I have succeeded in keeping my weight under control with a minimum amount of discomfort.

The strategy for feeding my body with 50 carbohydrates a day is simple. I prepare for the battle with my own carb-controlled delicious dishes. I always have plenty around, ready to please my cravings for food at any moment. It's packaged, in my refrigerator and ready for home or for "take out" when I have to go out of my domain.

If I wish for something sweet I grab one of my celebrated flaxseed meal muffins, or a small bowl of low carb ice cream with berries, or an ice cream bar, or perhaps before bed an Atkins low carb bar. There are lots of choices.

If I wish for something salty I reach for stuff like guacamole, hummus, lavash bread, chicharrones, nuts, meat casseroles or soups. I keep discovering many more items that I can add to my cooking routine every day.

I can find in my local supermarkets a growing supply of low-carb products, though they are a little pricey. There are also a few specialized low-carb stores near my house and lots of low-carb products can be purchased online and delivered to my home.

The Smartphone Application Revisited

In our test program, some of the participants that tried the "50 Carbs program" did very well but others did not lost the weight as expected. After reviewing every case I realized that one of the main problems related to the incorrect way they used the app. It seems like they did not learn how to run the program properly, and they became frustrated with the process. It can get tricky; I remember spending some time learning how to operate it.

Why it mattered

The app became the most important tool for me because it gave me a visual way to tell my progress. I compare it to the gauges in a car's dashboard. Without them I couldn't tell how fast I was going, how much fuel I have or other critical information.

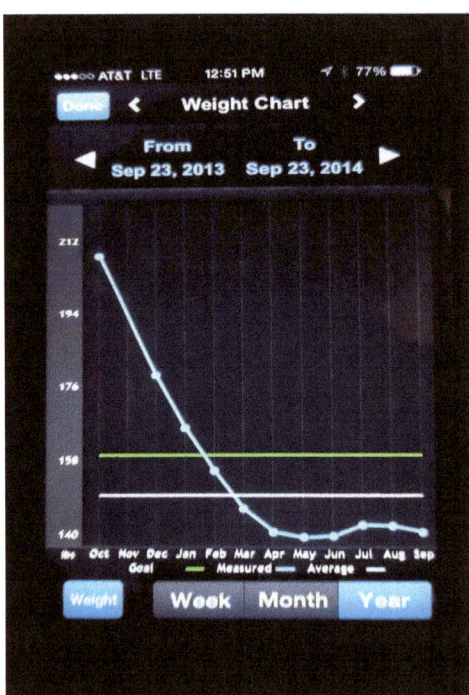

This picture, taken from the screen of my smartphone, is the graphic chart of my journey for one year. If you look in detail you can tell how much and when my weight dropped. I could even tell what I ate - every meal, any day during the diet.

This was for me the ultimate judge. To get this graphic I had to weight my self every morning and enter the results.

This is the reason I put so much emphasis on mastering the use of the app. I cannot tell you how much it helped me. It kept me informed during the whole journey and gave me a sense of complete control over the process.

The app that I used for my program is called "Diabetes App", I found it in the Apple store for the iPhone platform. There are many other apps as good as this one, as well as many for the Android platform.

50 Carbs

Remember, you don't have to be diabetic to use this app. I just took advantage of the "Carbs" feature to keep an accurate daily count of my carbs.

This app has a bank of over 200,000 food items, Once you know how, it's easy to add new products. You can enter your own recipes and add them to your tab with one click instead of having to list every item in your dish every time.

Sometimes it might feel overwhelming when you have to select stuff like chicken, ham or other types of meat. You'll find hundreds of choices (fried, breaded, baked, stewed, leg, thigh, breast, row, skin, skinless, portion sizes etc.). The same problem appears in lots of other products like fruits and vegetables. Remember once you find the correct choices send them to the "favorites" menu on your app. Then you can quickly locate them and with one click add them to your daily carb tab. It gets a little tricky until you get familiar with the process. This is where most of the early participants got confused and lost their patience.

Other features offered in the app became very helpful for the 50 Carbs program, like the weight feature to keep track of your weight.

For a quick refresher, please review the information in chapter 8 to explore the different features of the app.

Chapter 20

No App?

Running 50 Carbs without the app

I've heard different reasons why using an Application to help track and measure the daily progress of the 50 Carbs plan can be difficult. I understand the challenges, and don't want anyone to become discouraged or abandon the plan before they see the benefits. Using the application is the best way to achieve the best results, but there is no reason that a modified approach won't get you closer to your health goals.

We are all different – we live different lives, have different jobs, families, responsibilities and goals. It takes time and discipline to fully master the different parts of the application. Of the two, time can be the bigger hurdle. You can still find success with 50 Carbs. As you become comfortable with the plan you will discover, as I have discovered, little tricks and routines that will give you the most bang from the time you do have.

For those who might find the use of the app hard to understand, or don't have the time to deal with it, the following method of running the 50 carbs concept could work for you.

No App? No excuses!

I realize now that I really only use a few food items to prepare all of my daily meals - stuff like eggs, lavash, some vegetables and fruits, my own flax seed muffins, steak, chicken, and fish. It's easy to remember the carb value of these ingredients, and that makes budgeting 50 carbs a day very simple.

The ultimate goal is to budget 50 carbs. If you prepare well, it should work the same as it works with the app.

I believe that if you correctly follow my advice it will save you a lot of time and frustration. You just need to get creative in negotiating your daily carb ration. Before you know it you will be preparing delicious low carb meals for yourself and looking fabulous and sailing smoothly through the world of 50 Carbs without the suffering that the maintenance stage often brings. It worked for me and it should work for you!

If you decide to try the 50 Carbs plan without using the app to manage the program make sure you're prepared to follow these steps.

First, refer to the table in chapter 16 to find out find how much weight you need to drop to meet your first challenge.

Second, stock your pantry and refrigerator. As you've seen in my snapshot I favor low carb bread, tortillas, pastries, candies, ice cream, selected vegetables and fruits, cheese, any kind of meats, cold meats, and snacks.

Building blocks

I build my meals every day by combining the products in my pantry and my refrigerator. Let's take a quick inventory of the items I have in my kitchen.

No App?

MY PANTRY

Spices
Thyme - salt - pepper - pepper flakes - oregano -rosemary - garlic salt dried onions

Flavorings/Sweeteners
Cinnamon powder -sugar-free cocoa powder - sugar-free coconut syrup
Splenda - sugar-free jams

Oils/Baking
Canola oil - olive oil - flax seed meal - baking powder

Bases/Sauces
Chicken bouillon - chicken broth - beef broth - tomato sauce - soy sauce- red wine

Staples
Canned tuna - canned beans - mole poblano- green salsa - red salsa

Beverages/Snacks
Coffee - diet sodas – nuts - bags of chicharrones - Atkins low carb bars

MY REFRIGERATOR

Meat and Fish
Chicken thighs - chicken breast - steak - ground beef - rotisserie chicken - beef for stewing – tilapia – salmon - halibut - bacon - sliced ham sliced turkey

Veggies

Onion – garlic – avocado - green peppers - red peppers – leaks – spinach – lettuce - serrano peppers – carrots – squash – chayote - broccoli - green beans – mushrooms - roma tomatoes

Fruits
Cantaloupe – blueberries

Beverages
Diet sodas - bottled water

Cheese/Dairy
Monterey cheese - feta cheese – eggs - whipped cream - cheddar cheese

Snacks and Treats
Sugar free Jello - low carb ice cream - ice cream bars - peanut butter- hummus - salad dressing

Bread
Lavash - Sangak bread (a must, 1 portion = 2 net carbs, delicious!

Let's talk some more about bread. The lowest low-carb regular bread I found is the multigrain type, and a slice starts at around 15 net carbs. Some other breads could go as high as 50 net carbs per slice! Instead of regular bread I use <u>Sangak</u> a middle eastern type of bread with only 2 carbs per serving.

For low carb tortillas the best choice for me is <u>whole wheat lavash</u> bread with 3 net carbs per serving. There are many other types of lavash that are easy to find in many markets, although the serving is around 8 net grams. It beats a slice of regular bread or tortilla, and it's great for wraps, soft tacos and for scooping up the sauces in my meals.

Variety

I like what I like, and you like what you like. There are many different items that you may see as essential to your preferred types of meals and snacks. Staples like cereals, milk and different types of snacks should be researched and understood as you fine-tune your meal plans. Remember, the key enemies to success are hunger and boring, bland food. Build you plans with this in mind!

You can get great information about the carb and nutritional content of different ingredients from many sources, and don't forget to check the labels on prepared and packaged foods that you will use to stock your pantry.

Here's a great place to look information on reading and understanding packaging labels.

English:
http://www.fda.gov/food/ingredientspackaginglabeling/labelingnutrition/ucm267499.htm

Spanish:
http://www.fda.gov/Food/IngredientsPackagingLabeling/LabelingNutrition/ucm268173.htm

Rules of thumb - Listen carefully!

Avoid all flour products like breads, tortillas, cakes, pastas, desserts. I use substitutions, and some are great!

Avoid most of the products that are not sugar free, like sodas, candies, and prepared snacks. I look for products low in carbs, (information on carbs and portion sizes are on the packages) or sweetened with Splenda or similar sweeteners.

I avoid some of the vegetables and fruits that are high in carbohydrates like bananas, corn, pineapple, potatoes, some juices, beans and rice. I only use a very limited portion (2 spoonfuls) when I have to.

Lucky for me all meats are practically free of carbs and most of the essential spices I use for injecting tons of flavor while cooking are carb-free as well.

I make sure that I always have a good supply of low carb food in my pantry and in my refrigerator. This is very important. Believe me, without them it's like going to the war without a weapon; for sure I'd perish in a few days.

It would be nice not to go over 1500 calories a day, but keeping a separate tab might complicate the matter. Use your common sense, and just keep tabs of your carbs for now.

Helpful Links

Here are a few terrific sources of information that can help you as you manage your carbs. They can be especially helpful if you don't have easy access to a scale or an app.
Use your hand as a portion estimator!

http://education.wichita.edu/caduceus/examples/servings/visual_estimates.htm

http://aka.weightwatchers.com/images/1033/dynamic/GCMSImages/PortionEstimator_Printable_013012.pdf

Chapter 21
Maintenance Mode

Let's Create!

So now we're in Maintenance Mode, where the things I've learned over the past year have become pretty consistent, and my dependence on my smartphone application is not as critical. Here's a look at my current routine, with some examples of how I manage my daily food intake.

On an average day I put together the following meals, using the stuff from my pantry and fridge.

My present Breakfast

3 scrambled eggs with two spoonful's of pinto beans	4 net carbs
3 bacon slices	0 net carbs
one portion of sangak bread or lavash	2 net carbs
2 spoonful green salsa	2 net carbs
2 cups of black coffee with Splenda	0 net carbs
half of my own recipe chocolate flax seed muffin	5 net carbs
Total	13 net carbs

As you can see this is a big breakfast. This meal can manage my appetite for a few hours before I get hungry again.

Mid-day and mid afternoon snacks

Most of the time I'll make myself a couple of taquitos using lavash as a tortilla. I stuff them with almost anything, like leftovers from breakfast, lunch or dinner. Other times I might eat a few chicharrones (pork rinds) with guacamole or treat myself to a little ice cream with a whole or half of one of my special chocolate muffins and coffee. It really depends what's available at the moment.

I estimated the carb value of this meal to be 5 net carbs

Lunch and Dinner

I usually eat a serving of my chicken or ground beef casserole or lasagna (using thin squash slices instead of pasta) that I've prepared in advance. Or I'll have a bowl of chicken soup, pepper steak, a piece of rotisserie chicken, steak, fish, pork. lamb with a side of vegetables or salad and obviously more lavash or sangak bread and for dessert a little bit of fruit or a few berries with whipped cream, coffee, perhaps a half of my muffins and sometimes a glass of merlot.

I estimate the carb value of this meal to be 15 net carbs

Before Bed

Sometimes I'll have half of a muffin (when I can control myself), or an ice cream bar, or a few pork rinds. There are many more options, but I end my day consuming around 50 carbs.

I go to sleep with my stomach feeling content because the food supply throughout the day was decent. I did not put myself through the misery of only having little or bland food to eat. It makes a big difference.

The first thing I do the next morning is step on my scale and weigh myself. I still get a feeling of intense suspense waiting for the results to be displayed.

Sometimes there's no movement in the scale for a couple of days, and I get worried. Then the next day the scale would register a drop of 3 or 4 pounds. Weird! It's one of nicest rushes I ever had. I feel so proud of myself.

Nothing beats the feeling of crossing the line, of reaching an unreachable goal, powered by your discipline and your willpower. To be rewarded with so many positive things – like extending your life for a few years, looking fantastic, driving back deadly illness like diabetes, high blood pressure, and high cholesterol… it's a very good deal, don't you think? This success is something you can appreciate even more if you pass the 60-year mark.

The Internet is your friend!

Just out of curiosity I recently explored a couple of social media sites - Pinterest and Tumblr. I was amazed to find hundred of awesome low carb recipes. One that caught my eye uses cauliflower instead of potatoes for mashed potatoes. That sounds like something I can work with and make it a great side dish for a steak. I know the more I look the more I'll find. Using these recipes and approaches as a foundation I can substitute my favorite seasonings to make them the way I like. You can do the same thing! Of course, we may find ourselves lost in the web, chewing up that precious time we all don't have enough of! Plan wisely and budget smartly.

Use Time Wisely

Many of us have families we take care of, and we all need to eat. This means we do one of three things: cook, eat out or order in! To me, cooking makes the most sense because I can control what happens. I can control what goes into the meal, what it tastes like, what it looks like and what it costs. Of course there are times where I go out to eat – business meetings, family gatherings, even a quiet night out with my wife. When I am home in my domain, I cook.

When I first started developing 50 Carbs, I spent countless hours researching different sites to gather as much information as possible. I spent another block of time working on my cooking skills, finding through trial and error the best ways to prepare my meals so they were both delicious and healthy.

As I become more comfortable with the plan, I set aside a few hours a week to prepare several meals that I package for use during the week. This to me is the most sensible approach, as I don't have to worry every day about finding the time and ingredients to prepare a full meal. With a variety of options already made, I can focus on adding the final touches – fresh veggies or fruit, a slice of Lavash or Sangak, a nice fresh glass of sugar-free iced tea, and a low-carb dessert to end the meal.

Not only do I save time and stress, but I really enjoy the whole cooking experience. Learning and exploring different flavors and techniques relaxes me and makes me happy, and boy does the house smell great!

So, to sum it up!

- Use the time you have to make the things you love.
- Prepare meals ahead, making enough to spread across the week.
- Make it interesting - don't be afraid to try new flavors.
- Portions ready to go make daily mealtimes a breeze. Just add the fresh!

- Keep your kitchen stocked with the basics, and you'll be ready to cook when you want to cook.
- No excuses!

Chapter 22

From a Friend

Fher Olvera, front man for Mexican Superstars Maná, philanthropist and activist:

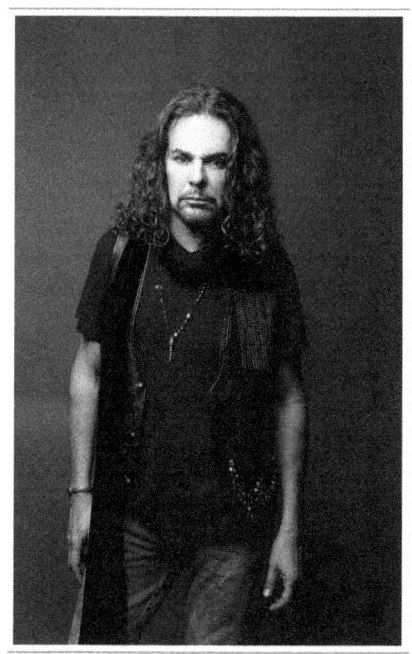

"José Quintana – my long-time friend who I call "Pepé", has been a key contributor to the success of Maná. We've worked together on many projects, creating and recording some great music over our 30-year friendship.

Pepé always loved food. I remember he would always wear a little "gordito" outfit – a little fat suit. Over the years he grew larger, and while he would try different diets he never quite stuck with any of them.

I hadn't seen him in a while, and when we got together in January of 2014, I was shocked – happily shocked. No more "gordito" outfit – my friend was now rocking a whole new skinny suit. He looked fantastic, happy and healthy. Seeing his transformation and hearing his story was inspiring, and showed me that there are ways to make positive changes in our life. I know so many people – friends, family and fans alike, who would find help, guidance and inspiration in Pepé's story. With obesity and diabetes high on the health concerns chart, the 50 Carbs plan that transformed my friend should find a place in every home, everywhere.

From a Friend

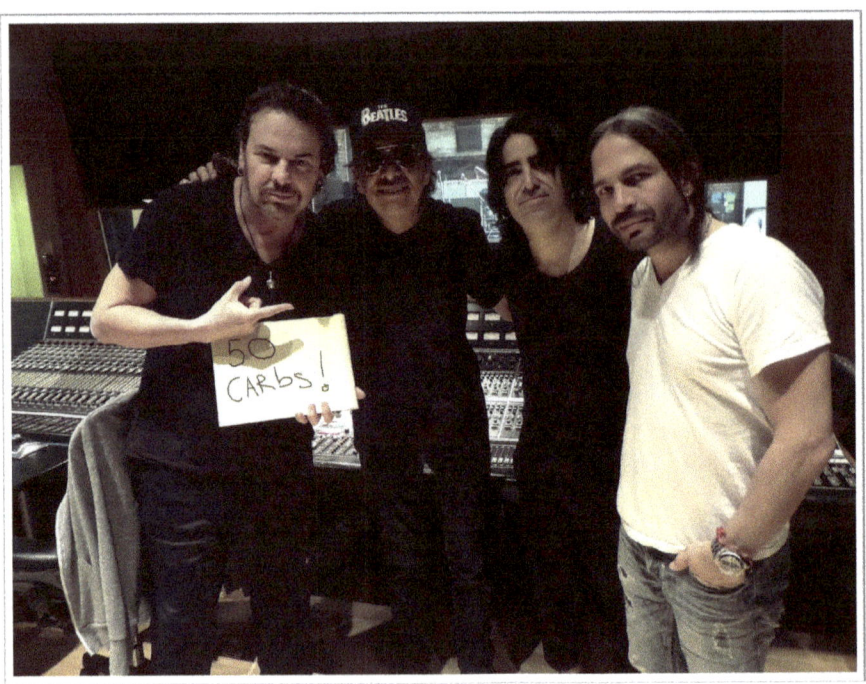

Maná – International Superstars from Guadalajara Mexico, have sold over 60 million albums worldwide. They appeared as guest artists on Carlos Santana's Supernatural album. While performing at an Inaugural event Maná was described as "the Rolling Stones of Latin America" by President Obama.

Chapter 23

From my Doctor

Michael D. Marsh, M.D.

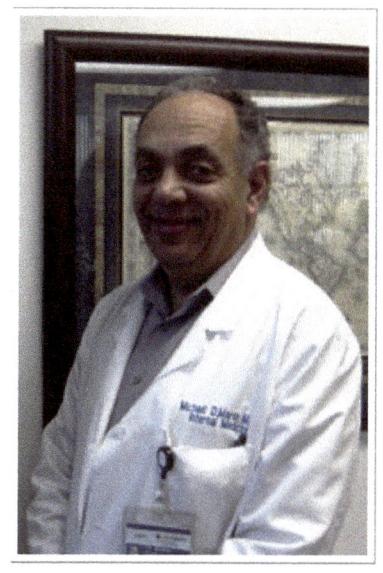

As a physician I meet and treat a wide range of people with a wide range of health related challenges. We are fortunate to live in exciting times where advances in science and technology help us live better, healthier and happier lives. Though we discover new ways to treat illness and disease, the best thing we can do for ourselves is to avoid those things that lead us to illness.

José Quintana has taken this simple and ageless advice to heart. I had been treating him for some time, helping him manage his diabetes and related issues that were gradually eroding his health and putting him at risk for potential severe problems as he aged.

Imagine my amazement when he came in to my office for an annual physical and review of his medications and treatment plans. The person I saw – and did not recognize at first – was a completely different man from the one who walked out of my office many months before. The physical transformation was dramatic. There was a slim, happy and energized guy where an overweight, unhealthy man once stood.

From My Doctor

During my examination, José shared his story about how, facing what he knew was a declining picture, he took charge of his health and forged a plan that would combine a realistic, statistically-based diet with an artistic and lively range of meals that were delicious, easy to prepare, and nutritionally sensible – what José calls "50 Carbs". With a primary focus on managed daily Carbohydrate intake, José turned what for many – including himself – can be a grim and sometimes unpleasant "DIET" into a healthy and delicious journey to better health.

The real joy came with the results of his blood tests. The key numbers – blood sugar, cholesterol… went from worrisome to wow! He went from the classic diabetic profile to a healthier person who had amazing control over his own health.

We have now moved from a multi-prescription regimen for managing his diabetes to a natural diet and exercise approach to maintaining health.

The "50 Carb" approach makes good sense, and goes after the key obstacles - hunger and boring meals - that cause many well-intentioned diet regimens to eventually fail. This sensible, managed approach to health and diet can be a great game plan for anyone who has been struggling to take charge of their own health. I am so pleased to see the change in José, and would be equally pleased to see these changes in everyone who suffers the sad effects of poor diet.

José

50 Carbs

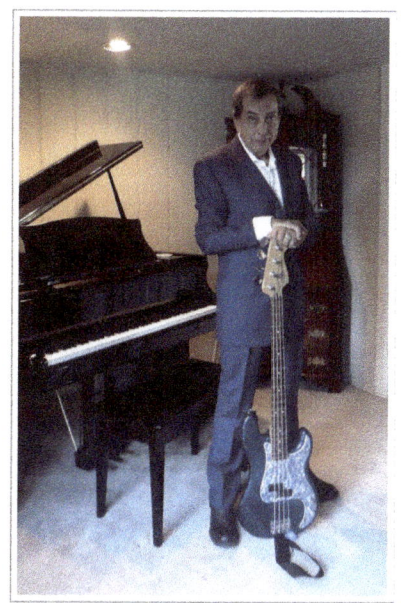

Like millions of others around the world, José Quintana found himself facing the unhappy prospect of declining health and quality of life from the effects of obesity and diabetes. 50 Carbs tells the story of José's journey from his early days as a child, through his adventures as a musician in Mexico, and on through his global career in the music business. Each chapter of his life fed his ever-growing love of food, and the ever-growing waistline that came with it.

Finally, José had enough. He knew that he needed to take a more active role in managing his health. He took the time to research various diet approaches and put together the 50 Carbs plan – a combination of tools, strategies and recipes that supported him as he went from obesity and diabetes to a slim, healthy and medication-free lifestyle. 50 Carbs provides a clear, low-stress approach filled with practical strategies, key tools and delicious recipes that can help others find their way to a healthier body.

50 Carbs – it just makes sense!

About the Authors

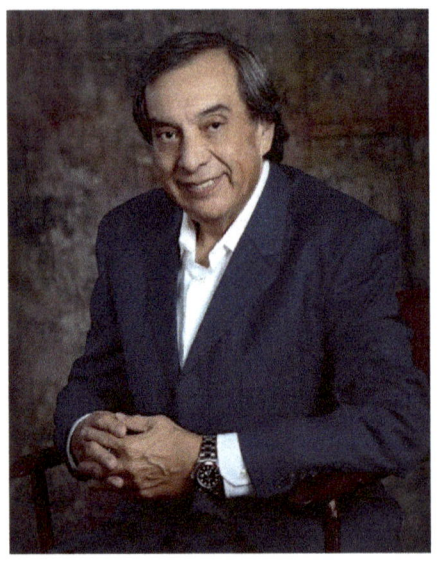

José Quintana has enjoyed an exciting and successful career as a musician and record producer. His passion, creativity and focus have contributed to the worldwide success of some of the most iconic artists in Latin Music. When he decided to take charge of his health, he applied these same traits to his second love - cooking. José's story is exciting, humorous and inspirational, and the lessons he has learned can help others find their way to a healthy and fulfilling lifestyle.

Michael Calderwood spent his "First Act" as a musician and writer, working across multiple disciplines from rock bands to live theater. "Act Two" was spent in an equally creative career working with a cast of engineers, designers, marketers and business innovators who represented the true blend of Art and Science. "Act Three" brings him home, where his passion for creativity and collaboration continues to grow and find new paths to explore.

Their blend of experiences, cultures, languages, skills and passions come together on the pages of 50 Carbs.

www.ingramcontent.com/pod-product-compliance
Lightning Source LLC
Chambersburg PA
CBHW040322300426
44112CB00020B/2847